GW01048633

# THE ITALIAN

# FOR COUPLE _Cookbook_

220+ Delicious Recipes
to make together!
Eat with your Partner
as in a Restaurant
with the most complete
guide about the
Italian Cuisine for two!

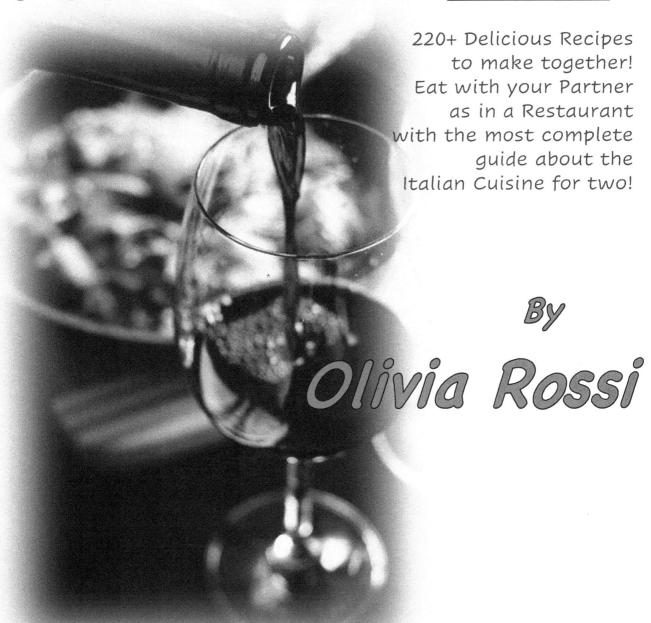

## By

## Olivia Rossi

# Table of Contents

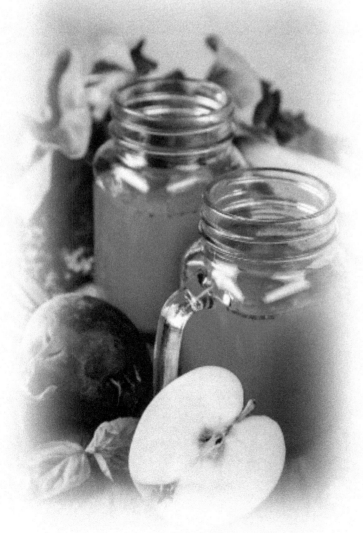

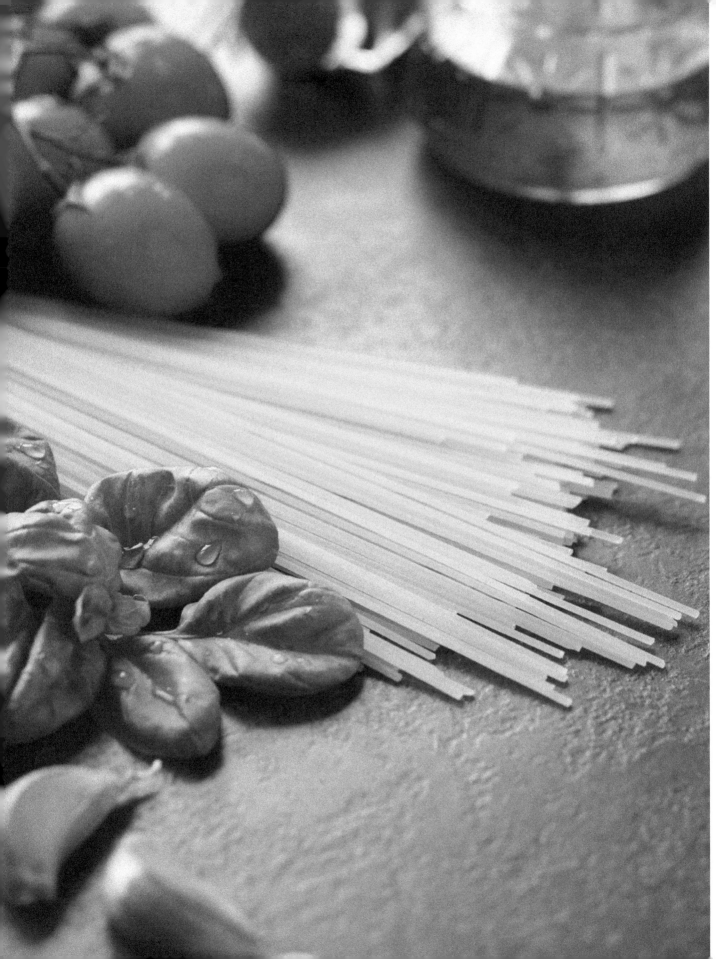

# Introduction

## The Italian Cuisine

Everyone knows Italian Cuisine: it is one of the most delicious and Healthy diet in the world! Everybody can follow Italian Diet: **children**, **older people**, **beginners**, **women**, and **men**! However, what is no better than a delicious <u>Italian dinner for two</u>?

In my life, I have often no time for cooking the right meals for my partner and me, so I wanted to create this fantastic cookbook to solve this problem to all my readers!
"The Italian Cookbook for Couple" was born for all **busy one** who want to have a fantastic lunch or dinners **with their partner**, without going crazy to find the ingredient and recipes for two different people! Indeed, this cookbook is a collection of 2 of my favorite books: "The Italian Diet for Women *Cookbook*" and "The Italian Diet for Men *Cookbook*": **the perfect combination you need!**
Become a real Italian: eat each dish tasting the ingredient mixes and stay HAPPY with your FAMILY!

You can choose many recipes with the best Italian ingredients such as:
- Cereals: bread, pasta, pizza
- Legumes: green beans, chickpeas, beans
- Proteins: milk, cheese, red meat, fish, light meat, seafood, nuts, extra virgin olive oil
- Fibers and vitamins: all of vegetables and fruits

Note - If you want to delight yourself: Add raw extra virgin olive oil to your food for the best experience ever! In the Italian Diet, it is important the quality of foods: foods must be fresh and, if possible, must be cultivated in Italy.

*Do you want to know The Best 220 Italian Recipes for Couple?*

## So, LET'S GO Together!

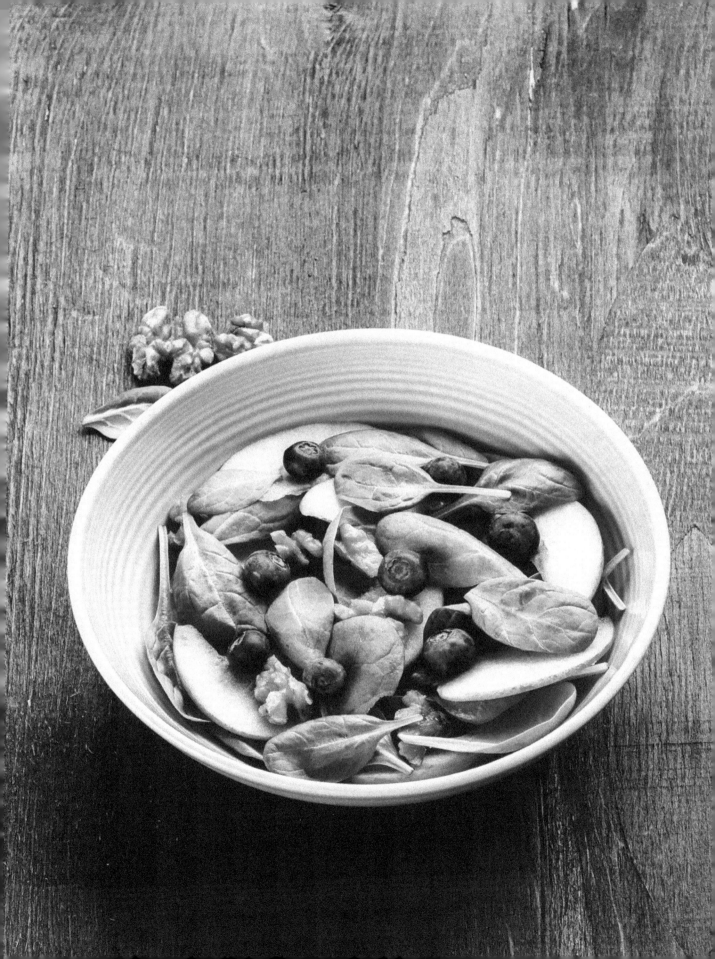

# Chapter 1.

# BREAKFASTS

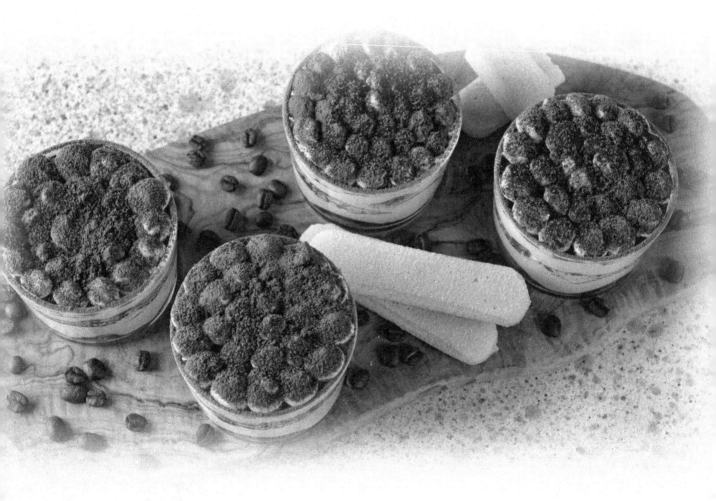

## 1) MUSHROOM OMELETTE WITH GOAT CHEESE

| | Cooking Time: 35 Minutes | Servings: 4 |
|---|---|---|

| Ingredients | | Instructions |
|---|---|---|
| ✓ 1 tbsp olive oil<br>✓ 1 small onion, diced<br>✓ 10 oz crimini or your favorite mushrooms, sliced<br>✓ 1 garlic clove, minced<br>✓ 10 eggs<br>✓ 2/3 cup half and half | ✓ 1/4 cup fresh chives, minced<br>✓ 2 tsp fresh thyme, minced<br>✓ 1/2 tsp kosher salt<br>✓ 1/2 tsp black pepper<br>✓ 4 oz goat cheese | ❖ Preheat the oven to 375 degrees F<br>❖ In an over safe skillet or cast-iron pan over medium heat, olive oil<br>❖ Add in the onion and sauté for 5 mins until golden<br>❖ Add in the sliced mushrooms and garlic, continue to sauté until mushrooms are golden brown, about 10-12 minutes<br>❖ In a large bowl, whisk together the eggs, half and half, chives, thyme, salt and pepper<br>❖ Place the goat cheese over the mushroom mixture and pour the egg mixture over the top<br>❖ Stir the mixture in the pan and cook over medium heat until the edges are set but the center is still loose, about 8-10 minutes<br>❖ Put the pan in the oven and finish cooking for an additional 10 minutes or until set<br>❖ Allow to cool completely before slicing<br>❖ Wrap the slices in plastic wrap and then aluminum foil and place in the freezer.<br>❖ To Serve: Remove the aluminum foil and plastic wrap, and microwave for 2 minutes, then allow to rest for 30 seconds, enjoy! |

## 2) SPECIAL STRAWBERRIES IN BALSAMIC YOGURT SAUCE

| Preparation Time: 15 minutes | Cooking Time: 180 minutes | Servings: 3.2 oz |
|---|---|---|

| Ingredients | | Instructions |
|---|---|---|
| ✓ 1 tbsp honey<br>✓ 1 tbsp balsamic vinegar | ✓ 1 cup sliced strawberries<br>✓ 1/2 cup yogurt | ❖ Mix all the ingredients in a bowl except strawberries. Put strawberries on top of each serving and refrigerate for 2-3 hours, then serve. |

## 3) GREEK SPINACH FETA BREAKFAST WRAPS

| Preparation Time: 5 minutes | Cooking Time: 5 minutes | Servings: 1 |
|---|---|---|

| Ingredients | | Instructions |
|---|---|---|
| ✓ Two eggs<br>✓ 4 Kalamata olives<br>✓ 1/2 cup spinach<br>✓ 1/4 cup feta cheese<br>1.5 tbsp butter | ✓ salt to taste<br>✓ One tortilla<br>✓ Black pepper to taste | ❖ Gather the ingredients. Heat the pan to medium heat. Add 0.5of a tbsp of butter to the pan. Scramble the eggs in a small bowl.Add in the rest of the butter chunks and salt and pepper. Add the egg mixture to the pan.Let the eggs cook for a moment, add in the spinach and mix till the spinach and egg are cooked. Put eggs over the tortilla.Top the eggs with the feta cheese crumbles and chopped Kalamata olives. |

## 4) ORIGINAL OMELETTE CUP OF CABBAGE AND GOAT CHEESE

| Preparation Time: 15 minutes | Cooking Time: 15 minutes | Servings: 8 |
|---|---|---|

| Ingredients | | Instructions |
|---|---|---|
| ✓ 2 cup kale<br>✓ 3 tbsp olive oil<br>✓ 1/2 tsp dried thyme<br>✓ One clove garlic | ✓ 1/4 tsp red pepper<br>✓ 1/4 tsp salt<br>✓ 1/4 cup Goat Cheese<br>✓ Eight eggs<br>✓ Black pepper | ❖ Preheat the oven to 350 F.<br>❖ Sauté the garlic in 1 tbsp of oil over medium-high heat, in a non-stick skillet, for 30 sec. Add the red pepper flakes and kale to it. Cook for a few minutes until the kale is soft.<br>❖ Whisk the eggs with pepper and salt in a medium bowl. Add the cooked kale and thyme to it.<br>❖ Take a muffin tin and brush 8 cups with the remaining oil. Put the mixture in it, topping with goat cheese.<br>❖ Put in the preheated oven and bake for about 30 min.<br>❖ Serve hot. |

**Nutrition:** Calories: 110 kcal Fat: 8 g Protein: 8 g Carbs: 3 g Fiber: 1 g

## 5) TASTY AND FLUFFY LEMON RICOTTA PANCAKES

| Preparation Time: 5 minutes | Cooking Time: 20 minutes | Servings: 6 |
|---|---|---|

**Ingredients:**

- ✓ 1.25 cup ricotta cheese
- ✓ Three eggs
- ✓ One lemon
- ✓ 3/4 cup buttermilk
- ✓ 2 tbsp sugar
- ✓ 1 tbsp baking powder 1.25 cup flour
- ✓ 1/4 tsp sea salt
- ✓ Olive oil

**Directions:**

- ❖ In a mixing bowl, whisk eggs and sugar.
- ❖ Add the buttermilk, salt, and ricotta cheese in it and whisk.
- ❖ In another bowl, mix flour and baking powder, then put it into the cheese mixture.
- ❖ Heat a large non-stick skillet. Spoon batter into the pan. Repeat with the remaining batter.

**Nutrition:** Calories: 245 kcal Fat: 9 g Protein: 12 g Carbs: 28 g Fiber:1 g

## 6) SPECIAL CAULIFLOWER FRITTERS AND HUMMUS

| | Cooking Time: 15 Minutes | Servings: 4 |
|---|---|---|

**Ingredients:**

- ✓ 2 (15 oz) cans chickpeas, divided
- ✓ 2 1/2 tbsp olive oil, divided, plus more for frying
- ✓ 1 cup onion, chopped, about 1/2 a small onion
- ✓ 2 tbsp garlic, minced
- ✓ 2 cups cauliflower, cut into small pieces, about 1/2 a large head
- ✓ 1/2 tsp salt
- ✓ black pepper
- ✓ Topping:
- ✓ Hummus, of choice
- ✓ Green onion, diced

- ❖ Preheat oven to 400°F
- ❖ Rinse and drain 1 can of the chickpeas, place them on a paper towel to dry off well
- ❖ Then place the chickpeas into a large bowl, removing the loose skins that come off, and toss with 1 tbsp of olive oil, spread the chickpeas onto a large pan (being careful not to over-crowd them) and sprinkle with salt and pepper
- ❖ Bake for 20 minutes, then stir, and then bake an additional 5-10 minutes until very crispy
- ❖ Once the chickpeas are roasted, transfer them to a large food processor and process until broken down and crumble - Don't over process them and turn it into flour, as you need to have some texture. Place the mixture into a small bowl, set aside
- ❖ In a large pan over medium-high heat, add the remaining 1 1/2 tbsp of olive oil
- ❖ Once heated, add in the onion and garlic, cook until lightly golden brown, about 2 minutes. Then add in the chopped cauliflower, cook for an additional 2 minutes, until the cauliflower is golden
- ❖ Turn the heat down to low and cover the pan, cook until the cauliflower is fork tender and the onions are golden brown and caramelized, stirring often, about 3-5 minutes
- ❖ Transfer the cauliflower mixture to the food processor, drain and rinse the remaining can of chickpeas and add them into the food processor, along with the salt and a pinch of pepper. Blend until smooth, and the mixture starts to ball, stop to scrape down the sides as needed
- ❖ Transfer the cauliflower mixture into a large bowl and add in 1/2 cup of the roasted chickpea crumbs (you won't use all of the crumbs, but it is easier to break them down when you have a larger amount.), stir until well combined
- ❖ In a large bowl over medium heat, add in enough oil to lightly cover the bottom of a large pan
- ❖ Working in batches, cook the patties until golden brown, about 2-3 minutes, flip and cook again
- ❖ Distribute among the container, placing parchment paper in between the fritters. Store in the fridge for 2-3 days
- ❖ To Serve: Heat through in the oven at 350F for 5-8 minutes. Top with hummus, green onion and enjoy!
- ❖ Recipe Notes: Don't add too much oil while frying the fritter or they will end up soggy. Use only enough to cover the pan. Use a fork while frying and resist the urge to flip them every minute to see if they are golden

**Nutrition:** Calories:333;Total Carbohydrates: 45g;Total Fat: 13g;Protein: 14g

## 7) ITALIAN BREAKFAST SAUSAGE AND NEW POTATOES WITH VEGETABLES

| Cooking Time: 30 Minutes | Servings: 4 |
|---|---|

| Ingredients | More Ingredients | Instructions |
|---|---|---|
| ✓ 1 lbs sweet Italian sausage links, sliced on the bias (diagonal)<br>✓ 2 cups baby potatoes, halved<br>✓ 2 cups broccoli florets<br>✓ 1 cup onions cut to 1-inch chunks<br>✓ 2 cups small mushrooms -half or quarter the large ones for uniform size | ✓ 1 cup baby carrots<br>✓ 2 tbsp olive oil<br>✓ 1/2 tsp garlic powder<br>✓ 1/2 tsp Italian seasoning<br>✓ 1 tsp salt<br>✓ 1/2 tsp pepper | ❖ Preheat the oven to 400 degrees F<br>❖ In a large bowl, add the baby potatoes, broccoli florets, onions, small mushrooms, and baby carrots<br>❖ Add in the olive oil, salt, pepper, garlic powder and Italian seasoning and toss to evenly coat<br>❖ Spread the vegetables onto a sheet pan in one even layer<br>❖ Arrange the sausage slices on the pan over the vegetables<br>❖ Bake for 30 minutes – make sure to sake halfway through to prevent sticking<br>❖ Allow to cool<br>❖ Distribute the Italian sausages and vegetables among the containers and store in the fridge for 2-3 days<br>❖ To Serve: Reheat in the microwave for 1-2 minutes, or until heated through and enjoy!<br>❖ Recipe Notes: If you would like crispier potatoes, place them on the pan and bake for 15 minutes before adding the other ingredients to the pan. |

## 8) GREEK QUINOA BREAKFAST BOWL

| Cooking Time: 20 Minutes | Servings: 6 |
|---|---|

| Ingredients | More Ingredients | Instructions |
|---|---|---|
| ✓ 12 eggs<br>✓ ¼ cup plain Greek yogurt<br>✓ 1 tsp onion powder<br>✓ 1 tsp granulated garlic<br>✓ ½ tsp salt<br>✓ ½ tsp pepper | ✓ 1 tsp olive oil<br>✓ 1 (5 oz) bag baby spinach<br>✓ 1 pint cherry tomatoes, halved<br>✓ 1 cup feta cheese<br>✓ 2 cups cooked quinoa | ❖ In a large bowl whisk together eggs, Greek yogurt, onion powder, granulated garlic, salt, and pepper, set aside<br>❖ In a large skillet, heat olive oil and add spinach, cook the spinach until it is slightly wilted, about 3-4 minutes. Add in cherry tomatoes, cook until tomatoes are softened, 4 minutes. Stir in egg mixture and cook until the eggs are set, about 7-9 minutes, stir in the eggs as they cook to scramble<br>❖ Once the eggs have set stir in the feta and quinoa, cook until heated through. Distribute evenly among the containers, store for 2-3 days<br>❖ To serve: Reheat in the microwave for 30 seconds to 1 minute or heated through |

## 9) EGG, HAM AND CHEESE SANDWICHES IN THE FREEZER

| Cooking Time: 20 Minutes | Servings: 6 |
|---|---|

| Ingredients | More Ingredients | Instructions |
|---|---|---|
| ✓ Cooking spray or oil to grease the baking dish<br>✓ 7 large eggs<br>✓ ½ cup low-fat (2%) milk<br>✓ ½ tsp garlic powder<br>✓ ½ tsp onion powder | ✓ 1 tbsp Dijon mustard<br>✓ ½ tsp honey<br>✓ 6 whole-wheat English muffins<br>✓ 6 slices thinly sliced prosciutto<br>✓ 6 slices Swiss cheese | ❖ Preheat the oven to 375°F. Lightly oil or spray an 8-by--inch glass or ceramic baking dish with cooking spray.<br>❖ In a large bowl, whisk together the eggs, milk, garlic powder, and onion powder. Pour the mixture into the baking dish and bake for minutes, until the eggs are set and no longer jiggling. Cool.<br>❖ While the eggs are baking, mix the mustard and honey in a small bowl. Lay out the English muffin halves to start assembly.<br>❖ When the eggs are cool, use a biscuit cutter or drinking glass about the same size as the English muffin diameter to cut 6 egg circles. Divide the leftover egg scraps evenly to be added to each sandwich.<br>❖ Spread ½ tsp of honey mustard on each of the bottom English muffin halves. Top each with 1 slice of prosciutto, 1 egg circle and scraps, 1 slice of cheese, and the top half of the muffin.<br>❖ Wrap each sandwich tightly in foil.<br>❖ |

## 10) HEALTHY SALAD ZUCCHINI CABBAGE TOMATO

| | Cooking Time: 20 Minutes | Servings: 4 |
|---|---|---|

**Ingredients:**

- ✓ 1 lb kale, chopped
- ✓ 2 tbsp fresh parsley, chopped
- ✓ 1 tbsp vinegar
- ✓ 1/2 cup can tomato, crushed
- ✓ 1 tsp paprika
- ✓ 1 cup zucchini, cut into cubes
- ✓ 1 cup grape tomatoes, halved
- ✓ 2 tbsp olive oil
- ✓ 1 onion, chopped
- ✓ 1 leek, sliced
- ✓ Pepper
- ✓ Salt

**Directions:**

- ❖ Add oil into the inner pot of instant pot and set the pot on sauté mode.
- ❖ Add leek and onion and sauté for 5 minutes.
- ❖ Add kale and remaining ingredients and stir well.
- ❖ Seal pot with lid and cook on high for 15 minutes.
- ❖ Once done, allow to release pressure naturally for 10 minutes then release remaining using quick release. Remove lid.
- ❖ Stir and serve.

## 11) Bacon Brie omelette with radish salad

| | Cooking Time: 10 Minutes | Servings: 6 |
|---|---|---|

**Ingredients:**

- ✓ 200 g smoked lardons
- ✓ 3 tsp olive oil, divided
- ✓ 7 ounces smoked bacon
- ✓ 6 lightly beaten eggs
- ✓ small bunch chives, snipped up
- ✓ 3½ ounces sliced brie
- ✓ 1 tsp red wine vinegar
- ✓ 1 tsp Dijon mustard
- ✓ 1 cucumber, deseeded, halved, and sliced up diagonally
- ✓ 7 ounces radish, quartered

**Directions:**

- ❖ Heat up the grill.
- ❖ Add 1 tsp of oil to a small pan and heat on the grill.
- ❖ Add lardons and fry them until nice and crisp.
- ❖ Drain the lardon on kitchen paper.
- ❖ Heat the remaining 2 tsp of oil in a non-sticking pan on the grill.
- ❖ Add lardons, eggs, chives, and ground pepper, and cook over low heat until semi-set.
- ❖ Carefully lay the Brie on top, and grill until it has set and is golden in color.
- ❖ Remove from pan and cut into wedges.
- ❖ Make the salad by mixing olive oil, mustard, vinegar, and seasoning in a bowl.
- ❖ Add cucumber and radish and mix well.
- ❖ Serve the salad alongside the Omelette wedges in containers.
- ❖ Enjoy!

## 12) OATMEAL WITH CRANBERRIES

| | Cooking Time: 6 Minutes | Servings: 2 |
|---|---|---|

- ✓ 1/2 cup steel-cut oats
- ✓ 1 cup unsweetened almond milk
- ✓ 1 1/2 tbsp maple syrup
- ✓ 1/4 tsp cinnamon
- ✓ 1/4 tsp vanilla
- ✓ 1/4 cup dried cranberries
- ✓ 1 cup of water
- ✓ 1 tsp lemon zest, grated
- ✓ 1/4 cup orange juice

**Directions:**

- ❖ Add all ingredients into the heat-safe dish and stir well.
- ❖ Pour 1 cup of water into the instant pot then place the trivet in the pot.
- ❖ Place dish on top of the trivet.
- ❖ Seal pot with lid and cook on high for 6 minutes.
- ❖ Once done, allow to release pressure naturally for 10 minutes then release remaining using quick release. Remove lid.
- ❖ Serve and enjoy.

**Nutrition:** Calories: 161;Fat: 3.2 g;Carbohydrates: 29.9 g;Sugar: 12.4 g;Protein: 3.4 g;Cholesterol: 0 mg

## 13) FIGS TOAST WITH RICOTTA CHEESE

| | Cooking Time: 15 Minutes | Servings: 1 |
|---|---|---|

**Ingredients:**

- ✓ 2 slices whole-wheat toast
- ✓ 1 tsp honey
- ✓ ¼ cup ricotta (partly skimmed)
- ✓ 1 dash cinnamon
- ✓ 2 figs (sliced)
- ✓ 1 tsp sesame seeds

**Directions:**

- ❖ Start by mixing ricotta with honey and dash of cinnamon.
- ❖ Then, spread this mixture on the toast.
- ❖ Now, top with fig and sesame seeds.
- ❖ Serve.

## 14) QUICK SPINACH, FETA WITH EGG BREAKFAST QUESADILLAS

| | Cooking Time: 15 Minutes | Servings: 5 |
|---|---|---|

- ✓ 8 eggs (optional)
- ✓ 2 tsp olive oil
- ✓ 1 red bell pepper
- ✓ 1/2 red onion
- ✓ 1/4 cup milk
- ✓ 4 handfuls of spinach leaves
- ✓ 1 1/2 cup mozzarella cheese
- ✓ 5 sun-dried tomato tortillas
- ✓ 1/2 cup feta
- ✓ 1/4 tsp salt
- ✓ 1/4 tsp pepper
- ✓ Spray oil

**Directions:**

- ❖ In a large non-stick pan over medium heat, add the olive oil
- ❖ Once heated, add the bell pepper and onion, cook for 4-5 minutes until soft
- ❖ In the meantime, whisk together the eggs, milk, salt and pepper in a bowl
- ❖ Add in the egg/milk mixture into the pan with peppers and onions, stirring frequently, until eggs are almost cooked through
- ❖ Add in the spinach and feta, fold into the eggs, stirring until spinach is wilted and eggs are cooked through
- ❖ Remove the eggs from heat and plate
- ❖ Spray a separate large non-stick pan with spray oil, and place over medium heat
- ❖ Add the tortilla, on one half of the tortilla, spread about ½ cup of the egg mixture
- ❖ Top the eggs with around ⅓ cup of shredded mozzarella cheese
- ❖ Fold the second half of the tortilla over, then cook for 2 minutes, or until golden brown
- ❖ Flip and cook for another minute until golden brown
- ❖ Allow the quesadilla to cool completely, divide among the container, store for 2 days or wrap in plastic wrap and foil, and freeze for up to 2 months
- ❖ To Serve: Reheat in oven at 375 for 3-5 minutes or until heated through

## 15) BREAKFAST COBBLER

| | Cooking Time: 12 Minutes | Servings: 4 |
|---|---|---|

**Ingredients:**

- ✓ 2 lbs apples, cut into chunks
- ✓ 1 1/2 cups water
- ✓ 1/4 tsp nutmeg
- ✓ 1 1/2 tsp cinnamon
- ✓ 1/2 cup dry buckwheat
- ✓ 1/2 cup dates, chopped
- ✓ Pinch of ground ginger

**Directions:**

- ❖ Spray instant pot from inside with cooking spray.
- ❖ Add all ingredients into the instant pot and stir well.
- ❖ Seal pot with a lid and select manual and set timer for 12 minutes.
- ❖ Once done, release pressure using quick release. Remove lid.
- ❖ Stir and serve.

**Nutrition:** Calories: 195;Fat: 0.9 g;Carbohydrates: 48.3 g;Sugar: 25.8 g;Protein: 3.3 g;Cholesterol: 0 mg

## 17) EGG QUINOA AND KALE BOWL

| | Cooking Time: 5 Minutes | Servings: 2 |
|---|---|---|

**Ingredients:**

- ✓ 1-ounce pancetta, chopped
- ✓ 1 bunch kale, sliced
- ✓ ½ cup cherry tomatoes, halved
- ✓ 1 tsp red wine vinegar
- ✓ 1 cup cooked quinoa
- ✓ 1 tsp olive oil
- ✓ 2 eggs
- ✓ 1/3 cup avocado, sliced
- ✓ sea salt or plain salt
- ✓ fresh black pepper

**Directions:**

- ❖ Start by heating pancetta in a skillet until golden brown. Add in kale and further cook for 2 minutes.
- ❖ Then, stir in tomatoes, vinegar, and salt and remove from heat.
- ❖ Now, divide this mixture into 2 bowls, add avocado to both, and then set aside.
- ❖ Finally, cook both the eggs and top each bowl with an egg.
- ❖ Serve hot with toppings of your choice.

## 18) GREEK STRAWBERRY COLD YOGURT

| | Cooking Time: 2-4 Hours | Servings: 5 |
|---|---|---|

**Ingredients:**

- ✓ 3 cups plain Greek low-fat yogurt
- ✓ 1 cup sugar
- ✓ ¼ cup lemon juice, freshly squeezed
- ✓ 2 tsp vanilla
- ✓ 1/8 tsp salt
- ✓ 1 cup strawberries, sliced

**Directions:**

- ❖ In a medium-sized bowl, add yogurt, lemon juice, sugar, vanilla, and salt.
- ❖ Whisk the whole mixture well.
- ❖ Freeze the yogurt mix in a 2-quart ice cream maker according to the given instructions.
- ❖ During the final minute, add the sliced strawberries.
- ❖ Transfer the yogurt to an airtight container.
- ❖ Place in the freezer for 2-4 hours.
- ❖ Remove from the freezer and allow it to stand for 5-15 minutes.
- ❖ Serve and enjoy!

## 19) SPECIAL PEACH ALMOND OATMEAL

| | Cooking Time: 10 Minutes | Servings: 2 |
|---|---|---|

- ✓ 1 cup unsweetened almond milk
- ✓ 2 cups of water
- ✓ 1 cup oats
- ✓ 2 peaches, diced
- ✓ Pinch of salt

- ❖ Spray instant pot from inside with cooking spray.
- ❖ Add all ingredients into the instant pot and stir well.
- ❖ Seal pot with a lid and select manual and set timer for 10 minutes.
- ❖ Once done, allow to release pressure naturally for 10 minutes then release remaining using quick release. Remove lid. Stir and serve.

## 20) EVERYDAY BANANA PEANUT BUTTER PUDDING

| | Cooking Time: 25 Minutes | Servings: 1 |
|---|---|---|

- ✓ 2 bananas, halved
- ✓ ¼ cup smooth peanut butter
- ✓ Coconut for garnish, shredded

- ❖ Start by blending bananas and peanut butter in a blender and mix until smooth or desired texture obtained.
- ❖ Pour into a bowl and garnish with coconut if desired. Enjoy.

## 21) SPECIAL COCONUT BANANA MIX

| | Cooking Time: 4 Minutes | Servings: 4 |
|---|---|---|

| Ingredients | | Directions |
|---|---|---|
| ✓ 1 cup coconut milk<br>✓ 1 banana<br>✓ 1 cup dried coconut<br>✓ 2 tbsp ground flax seed | ✓ 3 tbsp chopped raisins<br>✓ ⅛ tsp nutmeg<br>✓ ⅛ tsp cinnamon<br>✓ Salt to taste | ❖ Set a large skillet on the stove and set it to low heat.<br>❖ Chop up the banana.<br>❖ Pour the coconut milk, nutmeg, and cinnamon into the skillet.<br>❖ Pour in the ground flaxseed while stirring continuously.<br>❖ Add the dried coconut and banana. Mix the ingredients until combined well.<br>❖ Allow the mixture to simmer for 2 to 3 minutes while stirring occasionally.<br>❖ Set four airtight containers on the counter.<br>❖ Remove the pan from heat and sprinkle enough salt for your taste buds.<br>❖ Divide the mixture into the containers and place them into the fridge overnight. They can remain in the fridge for up to 3 days.<br>❖ Before you set this tasty mixture in the microwave to heat up, you need to let it thaw on the counter for a bit. |

## 22) RASPBERRY AND LEMON MUFFINS WITH OLIVE OIL

| | Cooking Time: 20 Minutes | Servings: 12 |
|---|---|---|

| Ingredients | | Directions |
|---|---|---|
| ✓ Cooking spray to grease baking liners<br>✓ 1 cup all-purpose flour<br>✓ 1 cup whole-wheat flour<br>✓ ½ cup tightly packed light brown sugar<br>✓ ½ tsp baking soda<br>✓ ½ tsp aluminum-free baking powder | ✓ ⅛ tsp kosher salt<br>✓ 1¼ cups buttermilk<br>✓ 1 large egg<br>✓ ¼ cup extra-virgin olive oil<br>✓ 1 tbsp freshly squeezed lemon juice<br>✓ Zest of 2 lemons<br>✓ 1¼ cups frozen raspberries (do not thaw) | ❖ Preheat the oven to 400°F and line a muffin tin with baking liners. Spray the liners lightly with cooking spray.<br>❖ In a large mixing bowl, whisk together the all-purpose flour, whole-wheat flour, brown sugar, baking soda, baking powder, and salt.<br>❖ In a medium bowl, whisk together the buttermilk, egg, oil, lemon juice, and lemon zest.<br>❖ Pour the wet ingredients into the dry ingredients and stir just until blended. Do not overmix.<br>❖ Fold in the frozen raspberries.<br>❖ Scoop about ¼ cup of batter into each muffin liner and bake for 20 minutes, or until the tops look browned and a paring knife comes out clean when inserted. Remove the muffins from the tin to cool.<br>❖ STORAGE: Store covered containers at room temperature for up to 4 days. To freeze muffins for up to 3 months, wrap them in foil and place in an airtight resealable bag. |

## 23) EASY COUSCOUS PEARL SALAD

| | Cooking Time: 10 Minutes | Servings: 6 |
|---|---|---|

| Ingredients | | Directions |
|---|---|---|
| ✓ lemon juice, 1 large lemon<br>✓ 1/3 cup extra-virgin olive oil<br>✓ 1 tsp dill weed<br>✓ 1 tsp garlic powder<br>✓ salt<br>✓ pepper<br>✓ 2 cups Pearl Couscous<br>✓ 2 tbsp extra virgin olive oil<br>✓ 2 cups grape tomatoes, halved<br>✓ water as needed | ✓ 1/3 cup red onions, finely chopped<br>✓ ½ English cucumber, finely chopped<br>✓ 1 15-ounce can chickpeas<br>✓ 1 14-ounce can artichoke hearts, roughly chopped<br>✓ ½ cup pitted Kalamata olives<br>✓ 15-20 pieces fresh basil leaves, roughly torn and chopped<br>✓ 3 ounces fresh mozzarella | ❖ Start by preparing the vinaigrette by mixing all Ingredients: in a bowl. Set aside.<br>❖ Heat olive oil in a medium-sized heavy pot over medium heat. Add couscous and cook until golden brown.<br>❖ Add 3 cups of boiling water and cook the couscous according to package instructions. Once done, drain in a colander and put it to the side.<br>❖ In a large mixing bowl, add the rest of the Ingredients: except the cheese and basil.<br>❖ Add the cooked couscous, basil, and mix everything well.<br>❖ Give the vinaigrette a gentle stir and whisk it into the couscous salad. Mix well.<br>❖ Adjust/add seasoning as desired. Add mozzarella cheese.<br>❖ Garnish with some basil. Enjoy! |

## 24) EGG CUPS WITH TOMATO AND MUSHROOMS

| | Cooking Time: 5 Minutes | Servings: 4 |
|---|---|---|

| Ingredients | | Directions |
|---|---|---|
| ✓ 4 eggs<br>✓ 1/2 cup tomatoes, chopped<br>✓ 1/2 cup mushrooms, chopped<br>✓ 2 tbsp fresh parsley, chopped | ✓ 1/4 cup half and half<br>✓ 1/2 cup cheddar cheese, shredded<br>✓ Pepper<br>✓ Salt | ❖ In a bowl, whisk the egg with half and half, pepper, and salt.<br>❖ Add tomato, mushrooms, parsley, and cheese and stir well.<br>❖ Pour egg mixture into the four small jars and seal jars with lid.<br>❖ Pour 1 1/2 cups of water into the instant pot then place steamer rack in the pot.<br>❖ Place jars on top of the steamer rack.<br>❖ Seal pot with lid and cook on high for 5 minutes.<br>❖ Once done, release pressure using quick release. Remove lid.<br>❖ Serve and enjoy. |

## 25) ITALIAN SALAD FOR BREAKFAST

| | Cooking Time: 10 Minutes | Servings: 2 |
|---|---|---|

| Ingredients | | Directions: |
|---|---|---|
| ✓ 4 eggs (optional)<br>✓ 10 cups arugula<br>✓ 1/2 seedless cucumber, chopped<br>✓ 1 cup cooked quinoa, cooled<br>✓ 1 large avocado<br>✓ 1 cup natural almonds, chopped | ✓ 1/2 cup mixed herbs like mint and dill, chopped<br>✓ 2 cups halved cherry tomatoes and/or heirloom tomatoes cut into wedges<br>✓ Extra virgin olive oil<br>✓ 1 lemon<br>✓ Sea salt, to taste<br>✓ Freshly ground black pepper, to taste | ❖ Cook the eggs by soft-boiling them - Bring a pot of water to a boil, then reduce heat to a simmer. Gently lower all the eggs into water and allow them to simmer for 6 minutes. Remove the eggs from water and run cold water on top to stop the cooking, process set aside and peel when ready to use<br>❖ In a large bowl, combine the arugula, tomatoes, cucumber, and quinoa<br>❖ Divide the salad among 2 containers, store in the fridge for 2 days<br>❖ To Serve: Garnish with the sliced avocado and halved *egg*, sprinkle herbs and almonds over top. Drizzle with olive oil, season with salt and pepper, toss to combine. Season with more salt and pepper to taste, a squeeze of lemon juice, and a drizzle of olive oil |

## 26) SPECIAL SMASHED EGG TOASTS WITH HERBY LEMON YOGURT

| Preparation Time: 4 minutes | Cooking Time: 15 minutes | Servings: 4 |
|---|---|---|

| Ingredients: | | Directions: |
|---|---|---|
| ✓ Eight eggs<br>✓ One lemon<br>✓ One clove garlic<br>✓ Two fresh basil leaves<br>✓ Four slices of bread<br>✓ 2 tbsp chives | ✓ 2 tbsp dill<br>✓ 2 cup yogurt<br>✓ 3/4 tsp salt<br>✓ 2 tbsp olive oil<br>✓ 1/2 tsp black pepper<br>✓ 4 tbsp butter | ❖ Boil eight large eggs for exactly 6 minutes and 30 seconds. Let sit in the ice bath for 2 min, then peel the eggs and set aside.<br>❖ In a medium bowl, mince one garlic clove, finely grate the zest one medium lemon, then juice the lemon. Finely chopped 2 tbsp fresh basil leaves, 2 tbsp fresh dill, and 2 tbsp fresh chives. Add 2 cup yogurt, 2 tbsp olive oil, 0.75 tsp kosher salt, and 0.5 tsp black pepper.<br>❖ Cut four crusty bread. Melt 2 tbsp unsalted butter in a large skillet. Add 2 of the slices and cook until crispy, for 2 min per side. Shift to a large platter. Repeat with the remaining.<br>❖ Place the yogurt and eggs on the bread. Drizzle salt and pepper and herbs with oil |

## 27) ITALIAN AVOCADO AND EGG BREAKFAST PIZZA

| Preparation Time: 5 minutes | Cooking Time: 40 minutes | Servings: 4 |
|---|---|---|

**Ingredients:**

- 1 Hass avocado
- 1 1/2 tsp lime juice
- 1 tbsp cilantro
- 1/8 tsp salt
- Four eggs
- 1/2 lb pizza dough
- 1 tbsp vegetable oil

**Directions:**

- Cut the avocado in halves using a spoon, but it's flesh in a bowl. Add the lime juice, cilantro, and salt. Mash well with a fork to form a smooth paste.
- Divide the dough into four equal pieces. Roll each piece into a thin 6-inch circle.
- Place one of the dough circles in the center of the skillet. Cook for 1- 2 min, until it is browned. Turn and cook another side until browned, pressing down with a spatula. Shift it to a plate and repeat.
- Apply 0.5 of the avocado mixture onto each cooked slice of dough.
- Fry eggs to desired doneness and place each one on top of a pizza. Serve immediately.

## 28) TURKISH MENEMEN RECIPE

| Preparation Time: 5 minutes | Cooking Time: 20 minutes | Servings: 3 |
|---|---|---|

**Ingredients:**

- 3 tbsp olive oil
- 4 cup tomatoes
- 1/4 tsp black pepper
- Three green peppers
- Four cloves garlic
- 1/2 tsp salt
- Three green onions
- Six eggs

**Directions:**

- Heat olive oil in a pan, preferably cast iron. Add the chopped onion and green peppers and sauté until tender.
- Add the tomatoes, garlic, and green onions and boil for 10-15 minutes, stirring regularly until cooked down. Sprinkle salt over it.
- Let it boil uncovered until the eggs are gently boiled for 8-10 minutes. Enable the egg whites to cook well with a spoon. If you like hard yolks, cook longer.
- Dress ground black pepper over it.
- Garnish with chopped green onion and mint leaves. Serve in the pan.

## 29) EASY AVOCADO MILKSHAKE

| Preparation Time: 10 minutes | Cooking Time: 10 minutes | Servings: 3 |
|---|---|---|

- 1 cup milk
- One banana
- One avocado
- 3 tbsp honey

**Directions:**

- Blend milk, avocado, banana, and honey in a blender until smooth

**Nutrition:** Calories: 246.7 kcal Fat: 11.6 g Protein: 4.5 g Carbs: 33.8 g Fiber: 5.6 g

## 30) ORIGINAL PUMPKIN OATMEAL WITH SPICES

| Preparation Time: 3minutes | Cooking Time: 3 minutes | Servings: 1 |
|---|---|---|

**Ingredients:**

- 1/2 cup water
- ½ cup dried oats
- 2 tbsp pumpkin puree
- ½ cup unsweetened almond milk
- 1/2 tsp pure vanilla extract
- 1 tbsp maple syrup
- 1/4 tsp pumpkin pie spice

**Directions:**

- Mix all the ingredients in a bow.
- Microwave them for three minutes.

## 31) LOVELY CREAMY OATMEAL WITH FIGS

| Preparation Time: | Cooking Time: | Servings: 3 |
|---|---|---|

| Ingredients: | | Directions: |
|---|---|---|
| ✓ 1 tbsp light butter<br>✓ 1 tbsp honey<br>✓ Five whole figs<br>✓ 1 cup rolled oats | ✓ 1 cup low fat/skim<br>✓ 1 tsp vanilla extract<br>✓ extra honey to drizzle | ❖ Sauté honey in melted butter and stir in figs. Set aside.<br>❖ Again, melt butter and sauté oats with a few figs and roast for five minutes.<br>❖ Mix in milk and vanilla and boil.<br>❖ Remove the pan from heat when the desired consistency is achieved.<br>❖ Mix roasted figs and oats and serve. |

## 32) ORIGINAL BREAKFAST SPANAKOPITA

| Preparation Time: 10 minutes | Cooking Time: | Servings: 2 |
|---|---|---|

| Ingredients: | | Directions: |
|---|---|---|
| ✓ 1 tbsp butter<br>✓ 4 oz Spinach<br>✓ 1 oz feta cheese<br>✓ Two green onions<br>✓ Four eggs | ✓ 1/4 tsp black pepper<br>✓ 1/2 tsp dill weed<br>✓ 1 oz cheese<br>✓ 1 tbsp chives | ❖ In a medium skillet, melt the butter. Add the dill, onions, and spinach, occasionally stirring.<br>❖ In a container, combine the feta, eggs, dill, cream cheese, and pepper. Transfer the mixture in a skillet over the spinach. Toss and cook for a few minutes.<br>❖ Serve and enjoy it. |

**Nutrition:** Calories:288 kcal Fat: 22g Protein:18 g Carbs:5.3 g Fiber: 1.8g

## 33) DELICIOUS STUFFED FIGS

| Preparation Time: 10 minutes | Cooking Time: 8 minutes | Servings: 6 |
|---|---|---|

| Ingredients: | | Directions: |
|---|---|---|
| ✓ 12 large figs<br>✓ 1/4 cup toasted walnuts | ✓ 3-1/2 oz Cambozola cheese<br>✓ honey | ❖ Fill the fig with Cambozola and put it in a baking tray.<br>❖ Bake in a preheated oven at 350 degrees for eight minutes.<br>❖ Drizzle some walnuts and honey and serve. |

**Nutrition:** Calories: 203kcal Fat:8 g Protein: 5g Carbs:31 g Fiber: 4g

## 34) VEGETABLE BREAKFAST BOWL

| Preparation Time: 10 minutes | Cooking Time: 50 minutes | Servings: 3 |
|---|---|---|

| Ingredients: | | Directions: |
|---|---|---|
| ✓ One breakfast veggie sausage patty<br>✓ One egg<br>✓ 1/2 oz cheddar cheese | ✓ ½ cup roasted veggies<br>✓ optional mix-ins: tomatoes, herbs, spinach, avocado | ❖ Bake veggies in a preheated oven at 425 degrees for 45 minutes.<br>❖ Crack eggs and add cheese.<br>❖ Mix them all and serve. |

**Nutrition:** Calories:420 kcal Fat:31 g Protein: 24g Carbs:12 g Fiber:1 g

# Chapter 2. LUNCH

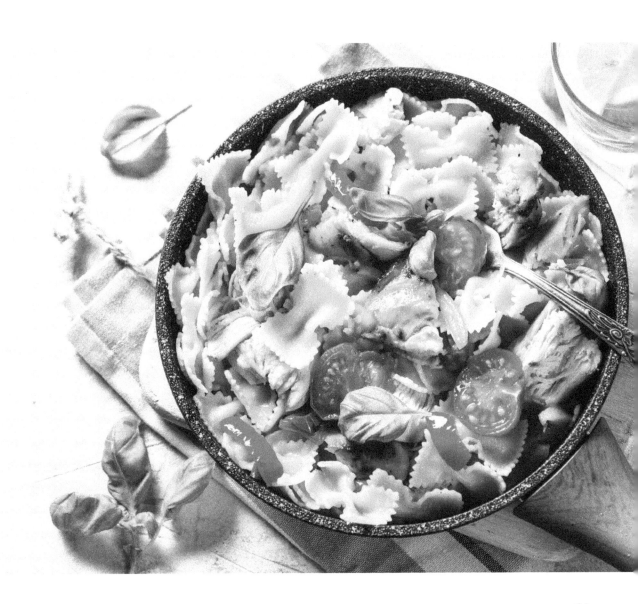

## 35) MOROCCAN-STYLE VEGETABLE TAGINE

| Preparation Time: 15 minutes | Cooking Time: 40 minutes | Servings: 5 |
|---|---|---|

**Ingredients:**

- ✓ ¼ cup extra virgin olive oil
- ✓ Ten chopped garlic cloves
- ✓ Two chopped yellow onions
- ✓ Two chopped carrots
- ✓ One sliced sweet potato
- ✓ Two sliced potatoes
- ✓ Salt
- ✓ 1 tsp coriander
- ✓ 1 tbsp Harissa spice
- ✓ 1 tsp cinnamon
- ✓ 2 cups tomatoes
- ✓ ½ tsp turmeric
- ✓ ½ cup chopped dried apricot
- ✓ 2 cups cooked chickpeas
- ✓ Handful fresh parsley leaves
- ✓ ½ cup vegetable broth
- ✓ 1 tbsp lemon juice

**Directions:**

- ❖ Sauté onions in heated olive oil at high flame for five minutes in a Dutch oven.
- ❖ Stir in veggies, salt, garlic, and spices. Mix well and cook for eight minutes over medium flame with constant stirring.
- ❖ Mix in broth, apricot, and tomatoes and cook for the next ten minutes.
- ❖ Reduce the flame and let it simmer for 25 minutes.
- ❖ Add chickpeas and cook for five minutes.
- ❖ Sprinkle parsley and lemon juice and mix well.
- ❖ Serve and enjoy it.

**Nutrition:** Calories: 448 kcal Fat: 18.4 g Protein: 16.9 g Carbs: 60.7 g Fiber: 24 g

## 36) ITALIAN-STYLE GRILLED BALSAMIC CHICKEN WITH OLIVE TAPENADE

| Preparation Time: 10 minutes | Cooking Time: 30 minutes | Servings: 2 |
|---|---|---|

**Ingredients:**

- ✓ Two boneless chicken breasts
- ✓ 1/4 cup olive oil
- ✓ 1/4 cup balsamic vinegar
- ✓ 1/8 cup garlic mustard
- ✓ 1.5 tbsp balsamic vinegar
- ✓ Three minced garlic cloves
- ✓ 1 tbsp lemon juice
- ✓ 1 tbsp chopped herbs of choice
- ✓ 1 tsp kosher salt
- ✓ 1/2 tsp black pepper

**Directions:**

- ❖ Combine garlic, balsamic vinegar, lemon juice, pepper, olive oil, herbs, salt, and mustard in a bowl. Add chicken and toss well to coat chicken.
- ❖ Set aside for three hours.
- ❖ Brush oil over chicken pieces and grill gates.
- ❖ Cook chicken on grill gates for ten minutes from both sides.
- ❖ Occasionally brush the chicken with marinade while grilling it.
- ❖ When marks appear over the chicken, shift the chicken to the grill gate's cooler side and cook there for 12 minutes.
- ❖ Again, shift the chicken to the heated side of the grill gate and cook for ten more minutes.
- ❖ Place the grilled chicken on a plate and cover to keep it warm.
- ❖ Serve and enjoy it.

**Nutrition:** Calories: 352 kcal Fat: 21 g Protein: 35 mg Carbs: 5 g Fiber: 1 g

## 37) ITALIAN LINGUINE AND ZUCCHINI NOODLES WITH SHRIMP

| Preparation Time: 20 minutes | Cooking Time: 20 minutes | Servings: 6 |
|---|---|---|

**Ingredients:**

- ✓ 2/3 cup extra virgin olive oil
- ✓ 1 lb shrimp
- ✓ Four minced garlic cloves
- ✓ Black pepper to taste
- ✓ 12 oz wheat linguine
- ✓ kosher salt to taste
- ✓ 3 tbsp butter
- ✓ Three zucchinis
- ✓ One lemon zested
- ✓ 1 tsp red chili flakes
- ✓ 3 tbsp lemon juice
- ✓ A handful of chopped parsley
- ✓ 1/2 cup shredded Parmesan cheese

**Directions:**

- ❖ Add salt, garlic, shrimps, pepper, and olive oil. Toss well to coat evenly. Keep it aside.
- ❖ Pour water into a pot and add salt to it. Let it boil and cook linguine in boiling water. Drain linguine and set aside.
- ❖ Heat olive oil in a skillet over medium heat and cook shrimps in it for three minutes from both sides. Shift the cooked shrimps into the plate.
- ❖ Melt butter in the same pan and sauté garlic, lemon juice, chili flakes, and lemon zest for one minute.
- ❖ Pour in pasta water in another pan and cook for three minutes. Add zucchini noodles and cook for two minutes with constant stirring.
- ❖ Transfer the noodles to the garlic mixture pan. Add linguine and cheese. Toss well.
- ❖ Pour in more of the pasta water to make a sauce of the desired level.
- ❖ Add shrimp, zucchini, salt, and pepper, and mix well.
- ❖ You can spread more cheese if you like.
- ❖ Garnish with parsley and serve.

**Nutrition:** Calories: 521 kcal Fat: 22 g Protein: 28 g Carbs: 52 g Fiber: 4 g

## 38) GREEK CHICKEN GYROS WITH TZATZIKI SAUCE

| Preparation Time: 10 minutes | Cooking Time: 8 minutes | Servings: 4 |
|---|---|---|

**Ingredients:**

- ✓ Greek Chicken
- ✓ 1 tbsp lemon juice
- ✓ 1/2 cup plain yogurt
- ✓ 1.25 tsp Italian-spiced salt
- ✓ 2 tbsp extra-virgin olive oil
- ✓ 1 cup Tzatziki sauce
- ✓ Four slices of pita bread
- ✓ Four chopped tomatoes
- ✓ 1/4 sliced red onion
- ✓ Tzatziki Sauce
- ✓ ½ halved cucumber
- ✓ ¾ cup Greek yogurt
- ✓ Two minced garlic cloves
- ✓ 1 tbsp red wine vinegar
- ✓ 1 tbsp chopped dill
- ✓ One pinch of kosher salt
- ✓ One pinch of black pepper

**Directions:**

- ❖ Marinate the chicken by mixing it with lemon juice, salt, and yogurt. Set aside for one hour.
- ❖ Heat olive oil in a skillet over medium flame.
- ❖ Add chicken without marinade and cook for five minutes from both sides. Transfer the cooked brown chicken to the plate.
- ❖ Mix all the ingredients of Tzatziki sauce in a bowl and set aside. The Tzatziki sauce is ready.
- ❖ Toast pita bread and place Tzatziki sauce, tomatoes, onions, and chicken pieces over pita bread. Wrap and serve.

**Nutrition:** Calories: 411 kcal Fat: 21 g Protein: 44 g Carbs: 10 g Fiber: 1 g

## 39) GREEK-STYLE CHICKEN MARINADE

| Preparation Time: 5 minutes | Cooking Time: 15 minutes | Servings: 4 |
|---|---|---|

**Ingredients:**

- ✓ 1 lb boneless chicken breasts
- ✓ ¼ cup olive oil
- ✓ ½ tsp black pepper
- ✓ 1/3 cup Greek yogurt
- ✓ Four lemons
- ✓ 2 tbsp dried oregano
- ✓ Five minced garlic cloves
- ✓ 1 tsp kosher salt

**Directions:**

- ❖ Mix all the ingredients in a bowl and set aside for three hours.
- ❖ Preheat the grill and grill chicken and lemon slices for 20 minutes from both sides.
- ❖ Slice the grilled chicken and serve.

**Nutrition:** Calories: 304 kcal Fat: 19 g Protein: 25 g Carbs: 14 g Fiber: 4 g

## 40) ITALIAN STYLE CHICKEN QUINOA BOWL WITH BROCCOLI AND TOMATO

| Preparation Time: 10 minutes | Cooking Time: 30 minutes | Servings: 3 |
|---|---|---|

**Ingredients:**

- ✓ Chicken
- ✓ 6 oz boneless chicken breast
- ✓ 1 cup Easy Roasted Feta and Broccoli
- ✓ 1/2 cup olive oil
- ✓ 1/2 tsp kosher salt
- ✓ Zest of one lemon
- ✓ 2 tsp dried oregano
- ✓ 1.5 tbsp lemon juice
- ✓ 1/4 tsp black pepper
- ✓ Two minced garlic cloves
- ✓ 1/2 cup Easy Roasted Tomatoes
- ✓ Quinoa
- ✓ 1 tsp kosher salt
- ✓ 1 cup dried quinoa
- ✓ Feta cheese to taste

**Directions:**

- ❖ Mix lemon juice, oregano, salt, olive oil, garlic, lemon zest, and pepper in a bowl.
- ❖ Add chicken and toss well. Set aside for one hour.
- ❖ Cook chicken in heat olive oil over medium flame for 15 minutes.
- ❖ Lower the flame and stir in tomatoes and broccoli and cook. Set aside.
- ❖ Add water and salt to a pot and bring it to a boil.
- ❖ Add quinoa and cook for ten minutes.
- ❖ Drain the quinoa and set aside.
- ❖ Add quinoa in a bowl, followed by the addition of chicken and veggies. Sprinkle salt, cheese, oil, and pepper.
- ❖ Serve and enjoy it.

**Nutrition:** Calories: 481 kcal Fat: 23 g Protein: 24 g Carbs: 45 g Fiber: 7 g

## 41) EASY CHICKEN PICCATA

| Preparation Time: 10 minutes | Cooking Time: 10 minutes | Servings: 4 |
|---|---|---|

**Ingredients:**

- ✓ 1.5 lb boneless chicken breasts
- ✓ One lemon
- ✓ 2 tbsp canola oil
- ✓ 1 tsp kosher salt
- ✓ 1 cup chicken broth
- ✓ 1 tsp black pepper
- ✓ 2 tbsp capers
- ✓ 3 tbsp butter
- ✓ 1/3 cup all-purpose flour

**Directions:**

- ❖ Mix salt, flour, and pepper in a bowl. Coat chicken with the flour mixture. Set aside.
- ❖ Cook chicken pieces in heated butter and canola oil over medium flame for five minutes from both sides. Shift cooked pieces onto the plate.
- ❖ Lower the flame and pour broth and add sliced lemon, butter (1 tbsp), lemon juice, capers, and cook for five minutes.
- ❖ Pour the sauce over chicken pieces and serve with cauliflower or noodles.

**Nutrition:** Calories: 381 kcal Fat: 20 g Protein: 37 g Carbs: 11 g Fiber: 1 g

## 42) ITALIAN CHOPPED GRILLED VEGETABLE WITH FARRO

| Preparation Time: 5 minutes | Cooking Time: 50 minutes | Servings: 2 |
|---|---|---|

**Ingredients:**

- ✓ 1 cup dried farro
- ✓ 1 Portobello mushroom
- ✓ 3 cups vegetable broth
- ✓ One sliced red bell pepper
- ✓ 1/2 sliced red onion
- ✓ 8 oz asparagus
- ✓ One sliced zucchini
- ✓ Olive oil as required
- ✓ 1/4 cup halved Kalamata olives
- ✓ One sliced yellow squash
- ✓ Kosher salt to taste
- ✓ 1-pint Greek yogurt
- ✓ Black pepper to taste
- ✓ 2 tbsp minced cucumber
- ✓ One chopped garlic clove
- ✓ 1 tbsp lemon juice
- ✓ 1 tsp chopped dill
- ✓ 1 tsp chopped mint
- ✓ Red bell pepper hummus
- ✓ 1/8 cup feta cheese

**Directions:**

- ❖ In a large pot, add broth and farro. Let it boil over a high flame.
- ❖ Lower the flame to medium and cook for half an hour with occasional stirring.
- ❖ Mix veggies with salt, olive oil, and pepper.
- ❖ Grill the veggies in a preheated grill until marks appear on them. Keep them aside.
- ❖ Whisk cucumber, salt, mint, dill, yogurt, lemon juice, and garlic in a bowl.
- ❖ Make the layers of farro, grilled veggies, hummus, olives, and cheese.
- ❖ Pour yogurt sauce and sprinkle mint and serve.

**Nutrition:** Calories: 140 kcal Fat: 6 g Protein: 4 g Carbs: 20 g Fiber: 5 g

## 43) QUICK PORK ESCALOPES IN 30 MINUTES WITH LEMONS AND CAPERS

| Preparation Time: 10 minutes | Cooking Time: 20 minutes | Servings: 4 |
|---|---|---|

**Ingredients:**

- ✓ Four boneless pork chops
- ✓ 1/4 cup all-purpose flour
- ✓ Eight sage leaves
- ✓ kosher salt to taste
- ✓ 2 tbsp chopped parsley
- ✓ 4 tbsp butter
- ✓ Black pepper to taste
- ✓ 1 tbsp vegetable oil
- ✓ 1/4 cup capers
- ✓ 1/2 cup white wine
- ✓ 1 cup chicken stock
- ✓ One sliced lemon
- ✓ 4 tbsp lemon juice

**Directions:**

- ❖ One each pork chops, place two sage leaves on both sides. Set aside.
- ❖ In a bowl, whisk salt, flour, and pepper.
- ❖ Coat pork chops with flour. Keep the sage leaves in place.
- ❖ Melt butter in a skillet over medium flame.
- ❖ Cook pork chops for five minutes from both sides.
- ❖ Clean the skillet and melt butter in it.
- ❖ Pour wine and add capers in skillet. Cook to concentrate the wine.
- ❖ Pour stock, lemon slices, and lemon juice. Let it boil for five more minutes.
- ❖ Place pork in sauce and cook for two minutes.
- ❖ Sprinkle parsley and serve.

**Nutrition:** Calories: 415 kcal Fat: 7 g Protein: 31 g Carbs: 14 g Fiber: 8 g

## 44) GREEK-STYLE CHICKEN KEBABS

| Preparation Time: 40 minutes | Cooking Time: 15 minutes | Servings: 6 |
|---|---|---|

Ingredients:

- ✓ 1 lb boneless chicken breasts
- ✓ 1/4 cup olive oil
- ✓ One sliced red bell pepper
- ✓ 1/3 cup Greek yogurt
- ✓ 10 tbsp lemons juice
- ✓ Four chopped garlic cloves
- ✓ Zest of one lemon
- ✓ 2 tbsp dried oregano
- ✓ 1/2 tsp black pepper
- ✓ One sliced zucchini
- ✓ 1 tsp kosher salt
- ✓ One sliced red onion

Directions:

- ❖ Whisk all the ingredients except chicken in a bowl. Add chicken and toss to coat chicken evenly. Set aside four hours for better results.
- ❖ Thread chicken, zucchini, onion, and bell pepper on the skewers.
- ❖ Grill the chicken, skewers on a preheated grill for 15 minutes, occasionally turning and basting with marinade.

## 45) Easy Salmon soup

| Preparation Time: 10 minutes | Cooking Time: 12 minutes | Servings: 4 |
|---|---|---|

Ingredients:

- ✓ Olive oil
- ✓ ½ chopped green bell pepper
- ✓ Four chopped green onions
- ✓ Four minced garlic cloves
- ✓ 5 cups chicken broth
- ✓ 1 oz chopped dill
- ✓ 1 lb sliced gold potatoes
- ✓ 1 tsp dry oregano
- ✓ One sliced carrot
- ✓ ¾ tsp coriander
- ✓ Kosher salt to taste
- ✓ ½ tsp cumin
- ✓ Black pepper to taste
- ✓ Zest of one lemon
- ✓ 1 lb sliced salmon fillet
- ✓ 1 tbsp lemon juice

Directions:

- ❖ Cook onions, garlic, and bell pepper in heated olive oil in a pot over medium flame for four minutes.
- ❖ Stir in the dill and cook for half a minute.
- ❖ Pour broth into the pot. Add carrot, potatoes, salt, spices, and pepper.
- ❖ Let it boil. Reduce the flame and let it simmer for six minutes.
- ❖ Add salmon and cook for five more minutes.
- ❖ Add lemon juice and zest and cook for one minute.
- ❖ Serve the soup and enjoy it.

## 46) RICH FALAFEL SANDWICHES

| Preparation Time: 20 minutes | Cooking Time: 10 minutes | Servings: 4 sandwiches |
|---|---|---|

Ingredients:

- ✓ 4 Pita Breads
- ✓ 1 cup arugula
- ✓ 1 tbsp lemon
- ✓ 1/2 cup tahini sauce
- ✓ 12 falafels
- ✓ One sliced red onion
- ✓ 1/2 cup tabbouleh salad
- ✓ Three sprigs mint

Directions:

- ❖ Spread tahini sauce followed by the addition of arugula and crushed falafels over pita bread.
- ❖ Add tabbouleh salad, mint, and onions over pita and drizzle lemon juice.
- ❖ Wrap the pita bread and serve.

Nutrition: Calories: 360 kcal Fat: 17 g Protein: 12 g Carbs: 44 g Fiber: 4 g

## 47) EASY ROASTED TOMATO AND BASIL SOUP

| Preparation Time: 10 minutes | Cooking Time: 50 minutes | Servings: 6 |
|---|---|---|

**Ingredients:**

- ✓ 3 lb halved Roma tomatoes
- ✓ Olive oil
- ✓ Two chopped carrots
- ✓ Salt to taste
- ✓ Two chopped yellow onions
- ✓ Black pepper to taste
- ✓ Five minced garlic cloves
- ✓ 2 oz basil leaves
- ✓ 1 cup crushed tomatoes
- ✓ Three thyme sprigs
- ✓ 1 tsp dry oregano
- ✓ 2 tsp thyme leaves
- ✓ ½ tsp paprika
- ✓ 2.5 cups water
- ✓ ½ tsp cumin
- ✓ 1 tbsp lime juice

**Directions:**

- ❖ Mix salt, olive oil, carrot, black pepper, and tomatoes in a bowl.
- ❖ Transfer carrot mixture to a baking tray and bake in a preheated oven at 450 degrees for 30 minutes.
- ❖ Blend baked tomato mixture in a blender. You can use a little water if needed during blending.
- ❖ Sauté onions in heated olive oil over medium flame in a pot for three minutes.
- ❖ Mix garlic and cook for one more minute.
- ❖ Transfer the blended tomato mixture to the pot, followed by the addition of crushed tomatoes, water, spices, thyme, salt, basil, and pepper.
- ❖ Let it boil. Reduce the flame and simmer for 20 minutes.
- ❖ Drizzle lemon juice and serve.

**Nutrition:** Calories: 104 kcal Fat: 0.8 g Protein: 4.3 g Carbs: 23.4 g Fiber: 5.4 g

## 48) GREEK-STYLE BLACK-EYED PEAS STEW

| Preparation Time: 5 minutes | Cooking Time: 55 minutes | Servings: 6 |
|---|---|---|

**Ingredients:**

- ✓ Olive oil
- ✓ Four chopped garlic cloves
- ✓ 30 oz black-eyed peas
- ✓ One chopped yellow onion
- ✓ One chopped green bell pepper
- ✓ 15 oz diced tomato
- ✓ Three chopped carrots
- ✓ 1.5 tsp cumin
- ✓ One dry bay leaf
- ✓ 1 tsp dry oregano
- ✓ Kosher salt to taste
- ✓ ½ tsp red pepper flakes
- ✓ ½ tsp paprika
- ✓ Black pepper to taste
- ✓ 1 cup chopped parsley
- ✓ 1 tbsp of lime juice
- ✓ 2 cups of water

**Directions:**

- ❖ Cook garlic and onions in a heated oven in a Dutch oven over medium flame for five minutes with constant stirring.
- ❖ Stir in tomatoes, pepper, water, spices, bay leaf, and salt.
- ❖ Let it boil.
- ❖ Mix black-eyed beans and cook for five more minutes.
- ❖ Cover the oven and reduce the flame. Simmer for 30 minutes.
- ❖ Squeeze lemon juice and mix.
- ❖ Serve and enjoy.

**Nutrition:** Calories: 187 kcal Fat: 3.5 g Protein: 9.3 g Carbs: 33 g Fiber: 9.6 g

## 49) TASTY JUICY SALMON BURGERS

| Preparation Time: 10 minutes | Cooking Time: 4 minutes | Servings: 4 |
|---|---|---|

**Ingredients:**

- ✓ 1.5 lb sliced salmon fillet
- ✓ 3 tbsp minced green onions
- ✓ 1 tsp coriander
- ✓ 2 tsp Dijon mustard
- ✓ 1/3 cup bread crumbs
- ✓ 1 tsp sumac
- ✓ 1 cup chopped parsley
- ✓ ½ tsp sweet paprika
- ✓ Kosher Salt to taste
- ✓ ¼ cup olive oil
- ✓ ½ tsp black pepper
- ✓ One lemon
- ✓ Toppings
- ✓ One sliced red onion
- ✓ Tzatziki Sauce
- ✓ One sliced tomato
- ✓ 6 oz baby arugula

**Directions:**

- ❖ Blend mustard and salmon in a blender.
- ❖ Shift the mixture in a container. Add all the spices, parsley, salt, and onions. Mix well and set aside for 30 minutes.
- ❖ Make patties out of salmon mixture and place in a tray.
- ❖ Coat all the patties with bread crumbs from both sides.
- ❖ Fry the patties in heated olive oil over medium flame for five minutes each from both sides.
- ❖ Drizzle lemon juice over the cooked patties.
- ❖ Spread Tzatziki sauce over the bun, followed by the layer of salmon, arugula, onions, and tomatoes. The salmon burgers are ready. Serve and enjoy it.

**Nutrition:** Calories: 365 kcal Fat: 19.5 g Protein: 40 g Carbs: 9.5 g Fiber: 1.6 g

## 50) SPECIAL BRAISED EGGPLANT AND CHICKPEAS

| Preparation Time: 20 minutes | Cooking Time: 55 minutes | Servings: 6 |
|---|---|---|

**Ingredients:**

- ✓ 1.5 lb chopped eggplant
- ✓ Olive Oil
- ✓ Kosher salt
- ✓ One chopped yellow onion
- ✓ One chopped carrot
- ✓ One diced green bell pepper
- ✓ Six minced garlic cloves
- ✓ 1.5 tsp sweet paprika
- ✓ Two dry bay leaves
- ✓ 1 tsp organic coriander
- ✓ ¾ tsp cinnamon
- ✓ 1 tsp dry oregano
- ✓ ½ tsp organic turmeric
- ✓ 28 oz chopped tomato
- ✓ ½ tsp black pepper
- ✓ 30 oz chickpeas
- ✓ Handful parsley and mint for garnishing

**Directions:**

- ❖ Sauté onions, carrots, and bell peppers in heated olive oil over medium flame for four minutes with constant stirring.
- ❖ Stir in salt, bay leaf, garlic, and spices and cook for one minute.
- ❖ Mix eggplant, chickpeas, tomato, and chickpea liquid.
- ❖ Let it boil for ten minutes.
- ❖ Remove the pan from flame and cover.
- ❖ Now, bake in a preheated oven at 400 degrees for 45 minutes.
- ❖ Sprinkle herbs and serve with any sauce.

**Nutrition:** Calories: 240 kcal Fat: 5.1 g Protein: 10.6 g Carbs: 42 g Fiber: 15 g

## 51) ITALIAN STYLE TUNA SALAD SANDWICHES

| Preparation Time: 5 minutes | Cooking Time: 0 minute | Servings: 4 |
|---|---|---|

**Ingredients:**

- ✓ 4 tsp red wine vinegar
- ✓ 4 tsp olive oil
- ✓ Eight bread slices
- ✓ ¼ cup chopped red onion
- ✓ 1/3 cup chopped sun-dried tomatoes
- ✓ ¼ tsp black pepper
- ✓ ¼ cup sliced olives
- ✓ 3 tbsp mayonnaise
- ✓ 2 tsp capers
- ✓ Four lettuce leaves
- ✓ 12 oz tuna

**Directions:**

- ❖ Mix wine and olive oil.
- ❖ Brush bread from both sides with oil mixture.
- ❖ Mix all the ingredients except lettuce and bread slices in a bowl.
- ❖ Place lettuce on each bread slices brushed with oil. Spread tuna mixture and cover with second bread piece and serve.

## 52) EASY SKINNY SLOW COOKER KALE AND TURKEY MEATBALL SOUP

| Preparation Time: 15 minutes | Cooking Time: 240 minutes | Servings: 4 |
|---|---|---|

**Ingredients:**

- ✓ ¼ cup milk
- ✓ 1 lb lean turkey
- ✓ Two slices of bread
- ✓ One chopped shallot
- ✓ ½ tsp grated nutmeg
- ✓ Two chopped garlic cloves
- ✓ 1 tsp oregano
- ✓ Kosher salt to taste
- ✓ 1/4 tsp red pepper flakes
- ✓ Black pepper to taste
- ✓ 2 tbsp chopped parsley
- ✓ ½ cup grated Parmigiano-Reggiano
- ✓ One egg
- ✓ 8 cups chicken broth
- ✓ 1 tbsp olive oil
- ✓ 15 oz white beans
- ✓ ½ chopped onion
- ✓ Two sliced carrots
- ✓ 4 cups kale

**Directions:**

- ❖ Soak pieces of bread in milk in a bowl followed by the addition of nutmeg, flakes, cheese, turkey, parsley, shallot, oregano, salt, egg, garlic, and pepper.
- ❖ Mix well using hands. Make meatballs out of the turkey mixture.
- ❖ Fry meatballs in heat olive oil in a skillet over a high flame. Keep the fried meatballs aside for a few minutes.
- ❖ Place beans, onions, carrot, kale, and broth in a slow cooker, followed by adding meatballs in broth.
- ❖ Cover the cooker and cook for four hours.
- ❖ Garnish with grated cheese, parsley, and flakes and serve.

## 53) SPECIAL SANDWICH WITH CHICKEN CAPRESE

| Preparation Time: 10 minutes | Cooking Time: 6 minutes | Servings: 4 |
|---|---|---|

**Ingredients:**

- ✓ 4 tbsp olive oil
- ✓ 1 tbsp lemon juice
- ✓ ¼ cup basil leaves
- ✓ 1 tsp minced parsley
- ✓ Kosher salt to taste
- ✓ Two boneless chicken breasts
- ✓ Black pepper to taste
- ✓ 10 oz sliced sourdough bread
- ✓ Eleven Campari tomatoes
- ✓ 8 oz sliced mozzarella cheese
- ✓ Balsamic vinegar as required

**Directions:**

- ❖ Add chicken pieces, olive oil, lemon juice, salt, parsley, and pepper in a bowl. Toss well to coat chicken evenly. Set aside.
- ❖ Grill the chicken on a preheated grill on a medium flame for six minutes from both sides.
- ❖ Toast the bread drizzled with olive oil.
- ❖ Sliced the bread into three pieces.
- ❖ Place chicken pieces, cheese, and tomato slices over each slice of bread.
- ❖ Sprinkle vinegar, oil, salt, basil, and pepper over the bread slices and serve.

## 54) AUTHENTIC MINESTRONE

| Preparation Time: 15 minutes | Cooking Time: 30 minutes | Servings: 6 |
|---|---|---|

**Ingredients:**

- 2 tbsp olive oil
- 1/3 cup shredded parmesan cheese
- Four chopped garlic cloves
- One chopped onion
- Two chopped celery stalks
- 1/3 lb green beans
- One diced carrot
- 1 tsp oregano
- Salt to taste
- 1 tsp basil
- Black pepper to taste
- 14 oz crushed tomatoes
- 28 oz diced tomatoes
- 6 cups chicken stock
- 1 cup elbow pasta
- 15 oz beans
- 2 tbsp chopped basil

**Directions:**

- Sauté onions in heated olive oil over medium flame for five minutes.
- Stir in garlic and cook for half a minute.
- Mix carrot and celery and cook for five more minutes with occasional stirring.
- Add oregano, beans, salt, basil, and black pepper and cook for another three minutes with constant stirring.
- Pour broth followed by the addition of tomatoes and let it boil.
- Lower the flame to low and let it simmer for ten minutes.
- Add pasta and kidney beans and cook for another ten minutes. Mix salt and serve after garnishing with cheese and bail.

## 55) LOVELY AVOCADO CAPRESE WRAP

| Preparation Time: 20 minutes | Cooking Time: 0 minute | Servings: 3 |
|---|---|---|

- Two tortillas
- Balsamic vinegar as needed
- One ball mozzarella cheese grated
- 1/2 cup arugula leaves
- One sliced tomato
- 2 tbsp basil leaves
- Kosher salt to taste
- One sliced avocado
- Olive oil as required
- Black pepper to taste

**Directions:**

- Place tomato slices and cheese, followed by avocado and basil. Over one side of the tortilla.
- Pour olive oil and vinegar. Drizzle pepper and salt.
- Wrap the tortilla and serve.

## 56) DELICIOUS CHICKEN SALAD WITH AVOCADO AND GREEK YOGURT

| Preparation Time: 10 minutes | Cooking Time: 0 minute | Servings: 4 |
|---|---|---|

- 1 cup plain yogurt
- 1 tbsp lemon juice
- One mashed avocado
- 1/3 cup dried cranberries
- Kosher salt to taste
- 2 cups shredded chicken
- Black pepper to taste
- 3/4 cup chopped celery
- 1/3 cup chopped pecans
- 1/2 cup chopped red grapes
- 1/3 cup chopped red onion
- 2 tbsp chopped tarragon

**Directions:**

- Whisk all the ingredients in a large mixing bowl.
- Serve as a salad and enjoy it.

## 57) EASY CHICKEN SHAWARMA PITAS

| Preparation Time: 10 minutes | Cooking Time: 30 minutes | Servings: 6 |
|---|---|---|

**Ingredients:**

- ¾ tbsp cumin
- ¾ tbsp coriander
- ¾ tbsp turmeric powder
- One sliced onion
- ¾ tbsp garlic powder
- ½ tsp cloves
- ¾ tbsp paprika
- 1 tbsp lemon juice
- ½ tsp cayenne pepper
- Eight boneless chicken
- Salt to taste
- 1/3 cup olive oil
- Pita bread
- Tahini sauce

**Directions:**

- In a bowl, add sliced chicken pieces, onions, cumin, garlic, cloves, olive oil, turmeric, paprika, lemon juice, salt, and coriander. Toss well to coat chicken evenly. Set aside for three hours in the refrigerator.
- Transfer the chicken pieces along with the marinade in a baking tray sprayed with oil.
- Bake in a preheated oven at 425 degrees for 30 minutes.
- Spread tahini sauce in pita bread and add baked chicken pieces. You can also add your favorite salad.
- Serve and enjoy it.

## 58) SIMPLE RED LENTIL SOUP

| Preparation Time: 10 minutes | Cooking Time: 45 minutes | Servings: 4 |
|---|---|---|

**Ingredients:**

- Four minced garlic cloves
- ¼ cup olive oil
- 1 tsp curry powder
- Two chopped carrots
- 2 tsp ground cumin
- One chopped onion
- ½ tsp dried thyme
- 1 cup brown lentils
- 28 oz diced tomatoes
- 4 cups vegetable broth
- 1 tsp salt
- 2 cups of water
- One pinch of red pepper flakes
- 1 cup chopped kale
- Black pepper to taste
- 1.5 tbsp lemon juice

**Directions:**

- Cook carrots and onions in ¼ cup of heated olive oil in a Dutch oven over medium flame for five minutes.
- Stir in thyme, cumin, garlic, and curry powder,
- Cook for half a minute.
- Add tomatoes and cook for another five minutes.
- Add pepper flakes, broth, salt, lentils, black pepper, and water in a Dutch oven.
- Let it boil. Cover the oven and lower the flame and let it simmer for 30 minutes.
- Blend a portion of soup of about two cups in a food processor and transfer it into the pot again.
- Mix chopped greens and cook for another five minutes.
- Remove from the flame and mix lemon juice and serve.

## 59) Tasty Scrumptious Breakfast Salad

| Preparation Time: 35 minutes | Cooking Time: 5 minutes | Servings: 4 |
|---|---|---|

**Ingredients:**

- Five eggs
- Two avocados
- One head romaine lettuce
- Two tomatoes
- Four clementine
- 1-pint strawberries
- One onion
- One cucumber
- One apple
- One peeled mango
- One nectarine
- 1/4 cup vinaigrette

**Directions:**

- Boil eggs in a pan. Turn off the flame. Let the eggs rest in hot water for 15 min.
- Cover spinach, avocados, tomatoes, strawberries, clementine, cabbage, peach, apple, nectarine, and cucumber in a large mixing bowl or on an individual platter. Sprinkle the vinaigrette at the tip.
- Take eggs from hot water; cool in ice water. Peel it and chop it. Spread the eggs over the salad.

**Nutrition:** Calories: 447.5 kcal Fat: 24.2 g Protein:13.4 g Carbs: 53.7 g Fiber: 15.6 g

## 60) SOCCA (FARINATA)

| Preparation Time: 10 minutes | Cooking Time: 20 minutes | Servings: 4 |
|---|---|---|

**Ingredients:**

- ✓ 1 cup chickpea flour
- ✓ One pinch salt
- ✓ ½ tsp cumin
- ✓ Black pepper
- ✓ 1 tbsp olive oil
- ✓ 1 cup of water
- ✓ 1 tbsp vegetable oil

**Directions:**

- ❖ In a cup, add chickpea flour, water, and olive oil. Season with salt, cumin, and pepper. Mix all ingredients. Set down at room temperature for two h.
- ❖ Preheat the oven to 450 degrees (230 degrees C). Place a cast-iron skillet in the oven until hot, 5 to 7 minutes. Gently remove the pan from the oven, brush the oil, and pour half of the mixture into the pan, tilting to ensure that it is evenly spread.
- ❖ Bake in a preheated oven bake it for 7 min. Switch the oven on and let it brown for 1 min. Turn off the oven and shift it to a plate. Do the same with the remaining mixture.

**Nutrition:** Calories: 145.6 kcal Fat: 8.4 g Protein: 4.7 g Carbs:13.8 g Fiber: 0.9 g

## 61) EASY BLUEBERRY LEMON BREAKFAST QUINOA

| Preparation Time: 5 minutes | Cooking Time: 25 minutes | Servings: 2 |
|---|---|---|

**Ingredients:**

- ✓ 3 tbsp maple syrup
- ✓ 1 cup quinoa
- ✓ One pinch salt
- ✓ ½ lemon
- ✓ 2 cup milk
- ✓ 1 cup blueberries
- ✓ 2 tsp flax seed

**Directions:**

- ❖ Wash quinoa in a fine sieve of ice water to extract bitterness when the water is pure and no stickier. Pour the milk into a pan over medium heat for 2 - 3 mins. Mix the quinoa and salt in the milk; boil over moderate heat once all of the liquid was being consumed, around twenty minutes. In the quinoa mixer, slowly fold the blueberries & add the apple and the lime juice. Serve quinoa mixture in 2 bowls; sprinkle 1 tsp linseed to eat.

**Nutrition:** Calories: 537.8 kcal Fat: 7.3 g Protein: 21.5 g Carbs: 98.7 g Fiber: 8.9 g

## 62) EASY ARTICHOKE AND SPINACH OMELETTE WITH CHEESE

| Preparation Time: 5 minutes | Cooking Time: 40 minutes | Servings: 8 slices |
|---|---|---|

**Ingredients:**

- ✓ 3 tbsp pesto
- ✓ 1/2 cup milk
- ✓ 12 eggs
- ✓ 1/2 cup parmesan cheese, shredded
- ✓ 2 tsp olive oil
- ✓ 14.5 oz artichokes, chopped
- ✓ Two garlic cloves
- ✓ 1 cup cheese
- ✓ 6 cup baby spinach
- ✓ 1/2 tsp kosher salt

**Directions:**

- ❖ Preheat the oven to 375 F.
- ❖ Take a bowl and put milk, eggs, cheese, salt in it, and whisk together. Dry the artichokes using a paper towel.
- ❖ Take a skillet and heat olive oil in it over medium flame. Sauté the garlic in it for half a minute and put 4 cups of baby spinach in it. Cook them until they become soft, and then add the rest of the spinach in it with artichokes and sauté.
- ❖ Add the egg mixture to the skillet and reduce the flame to medium-low. Cook the eggs for 1 minute without stirring.
- ❖ Once the eggs are cooked, stir it to mix well and top with leftover whole artichokes. Put the skillet in the preheated oven.
- ❖ Bake for about 20 minutes or until its edges start to turn brown and puffed from the top. Take out of the oven and put the pesto on it, and sprinkle with cheese. Bake for five more minutes or until the cheese melts, and a frittata is cooked thoroughly.
- ❖ Sprinkle the black pepper and fresh basil on top.

**Nutrition:** Calories: 234 kcal Fat: 16 g Protein: 16 g Carbs: 6 g Fiber: 2 g

## 63) SPECIAL STRAWBERRIES IN BALSAMIC YOGURT SAUCE

| Preparation Time: 15 minutes | Cooking Time: 180 minutes | Servings: 3.2 oz |
|---|---|---|

| Ingredients: | Directions: |
|---|---|
| ✓ 1 tbsp honey <br> ✓ 1 tbsp balsamic vinegar <br> ✓ 1 cup sliced strawberries <br> ✓ 1/2 cup yogurt | ❖ Mix all the ingredients in a bowl except strawberries. Put strawberries on top of each serving and refrigerate for 2-3 hours, then serve. |

Nutrition: Calories: 51 kcal Fat: g Protein:3 g Carbs: 9 g Fiber:1 g

## 64) GREEK SPINACH FETA BREAKFAST WRAPS

| Preparation Time: 5 minutes | Cooking Time: 5 minutes | Servings: 1 |
|---|---|---|

| Ingredients: | Directions: |
|---|---|
| ✓ Two eggs <br> ✓ 4 Kalamata olives <br> ✓ 1/2 cup spinach <br> ✓ 1/4 cup feta cheese <br> 1.5 tbsp butter <br> ✓ salt to taste <br> ✓ One tortilla <br> ✓ Black pepper to taste | ❖ Gather the ingredients. Heat the pan to medium heat. Add 0.5of a tbsp of butter to the pan. Scramble the eggs in a small bowl.Add in the rest of the butter chunks and salt and pepper. Add the egg mixture to the pan.Let the eggs cook for a moment, add in the spinach and mix till the spinach and egg are cooked. Put eggs over the tortilla.Top the eggs with the feta cheese crumbles and chopped Kalamata olives. |

Nutrition: Calories:399 kcal Fat: 22.9 g Protein: 19.6 g Carbs: 29.2 g Fiber: 2.3 g

## 65) ORIGINAL OMELETTE CUP OF CABBAGE AND GOAT CHEESE

| Preparation Time: 15 minutes | Cooking Time: 15 minutes | Servings: 8 |
|---|---|---|

| Ingredients: | Directions: |
|---|---|
| ✓ 2 cup kale <br> ✓ 3 tbsp olive oil <br> ✓ 1/2 tsp dried thyme <br> ✓ One clove garlic <br> ✓ 1/4 tsp red pepper <br> ✓ 1/4 tsp salt <br> ✓ 1/4 cup Goat Cheese <br> ✓ Eight eggs <br> ✓ Black pepper | ❖ Preheat the oven to 350 F. <br> ❖ Sauté the garlic in 1 tbsp of oil over medium-high heat, in a non-stick skillet, for 30 sec. Add the red pepper flakes and kale to it. Cook for a few minutes until the kale is soft. <br> ❖ Whisk the eggs with pepper and salt in a medium bowl. Add the cooked kale and thyme to it. <br> ❖ Take a muffin tin and brush 8 cups with the remaining oil. Put the mixture in it, topping with goat cheese. <br> ❖ Put in the preheated oven and bake for about 30 min. <br> ❖ Serve hot. |

## 66) TASTY AND FLUFFY LEMON RICOTTA PANCAKES

| Preparation Time: 5 minutes | Cooking Time: 20 minutes | Servings: 6 |
|---|---|---|

| Ingredients: | Directions: |
|---|---|
| ✓ 1.25 cup ricotta cheese <br> ✓ Three eggs <br> ✓ One lemon <br> ✓ 3/4 cup buttermilk <br> ✓ 2 tbsp sugar <br> ✓ 1 tbsp baking powder 1.25 cup flour <br> ✓ 1/4 tsp sea salt <br> ✓ Olive oil | ❖ In a mixing bowl, whisk eggs and sugar. <br> ❖ Add the buttermilk, salt, and ricotta cheese in it and whisk. <br> ❖ In another bowl, mix flour and baking powder, then put it into the cheese mixture. <br> ❖ Heat a large non-stick skillet. Spoon batter into the pan. Repeat with the remaining batter. |

## 67) GREEK-STYLE COUSCOUS SALAD

| Preparation Time: 10 minutes | Cooking Time: 0 minute | Servings: 2 |
|---|---|---|

**Ingredients:**

- ¼ cup of low sodium feta cheese
- Three cups of cooked couscous.
- One cup of cherry tomatoes
- One chopped scallion, green & white parts.
- One Eng. Diced cucumber.
- Half a cup of black olives.
- 2 tbsp of fresh chopped parsley.
- One tbsp of fresh lemon juice.
- 2 tbsp of balsamic vinegar

**Directions:**

- Mix all the ingredients in a large bowl.
- Top it with the feta cheese & the salad is ready to serve

## 68) GERMAN BRAISED CABBAGE

| Preparation Time: 15-20 min | Cooking Time: 15 min | Servings: 1 |
|---|---|---|

**Ingredients:**

- 1 tbsp of olive oil
- One-fourth chopped sweet onion.
- Five cups of shredded red cabbage.
- One pear, peeled & chopped
- 3 tbsp of vinegar.
- Half tsp dry mustard.
- One tbsp of sugar.
- Half tsp caraway seeds.

**Directions:**

- Heat olive oil on moderate heat in a frying pan.
- Add cabbage, onion & pear. sauté till tendered for 10 min.
- Stir together vinegar, caraway seed sugar & mustard in a bowl.
- Combine cabbage and vinegar mixture and stir.
- Cover for 5 min.
- Now Serve hot.

## 69) EASY VIBRANT CARROT SOUP

| Preparation Time: 10 minutes | Cooking Time: 20-25 minutes | Servings: 1-2 |
|---|---|---|

**Ingredients:**

- 1 tbsp of olive oil
- Half chopped onion.
- 2 tsp of fresh ginger.
- One tsp of fresh minced garlic
- 4 cups of water
- Three chopped carrots.
- 1 tsp turmeric powder.
- Half cup of coconut milk
- One tbsp of fresh chopped cilantro

**Directions:**

- Heat the olive oil in a saucepan on medium heat.
- Sauté onion, garlic & ginger till softened 3 min.
- Stir in water, carrots & turmeric. Bring a boil & reduce heat and simmer till the carrots are tendered (20 min).
- Transfer soup in a blender along with coconut milk and pulse until soup becomes smooth.
- Serve the soup topped with cilantro.

**Nutrition:** Calories: 113, kcal Fat: 10 g Protein: 2 g Carbs: 8 g Fiber: 2g

## 70) SPECIAL BREAKFAST SANDWICH WITH OPEN BAGEL

| Preparation Time: 10 minutes | Cooking Time: 10-15 minutes | Servings: 2 |
|---|---|---|

**Ingredients:**

- ✓ one halved multigrain bagel.
- ✓ Two tbsp divided cream cheese.
- ✓ Two slices of tomato
- ✓ One slice of red onion
- ✓ black pepper
- ✓ One cup of microgreens.

**Directions:**

- ❖ Light toast bagel in an oven or toaster.
- ❖ Spread one tbsp of cheese on each bagel halves.
- ❖ Top each half with one tomato slice & a couple of onion rings and season with black pepper.
- ❖ Now top each half with a half cup of microgreens. Now it is ready to serve.

**Nutrition:** Calories: 164, kcal Fat: 6g, Protein: 6g: Carbs: 23g: Fiber: 3g

## 71) ITALIAN BLACK-EYED PEAS SALAD

| Preparation Time: 10-15 minutes | Cooking Time: 15-20 minutes | Servings: 1 |
|---|---|---|

**Ingredients:**

- ✓ One and a half cups black-eyed peas.
- ✓ Half tsp of salt.
- ✓ 3/4 cup of chopped bell pepper.
- ✓ Half tsp of freshly ground black pepper
- ✓ Half cup chopped celery.
- ✓ 1/4 cup of olive oil.
- ✓ 1 tbsp of sugar.
- ✓ One clove of minced garlic.
- ✓ 2 tbsp of vinegar.

**Directions:**

- ❖ Combine peas, celery, green bell pepper & onion in a bowl and mix.
- ❖ Add oil, salt, sugar, vinegar, garlic, and black pepper in a bowl and mix with a fork.
- ❖ Pour this dressing over vegetables.
- ❖ Mix well.
- ❖ Add hot sauce according to taste.
- ❖ Toss to combine and put for a whole night.
- ❖ The dish is ready to serve.

**Nutrition:** Calories: 324 kcal Fat: 11 g Protein: 5 g Carbs: 17 g Fiber: 4 g

## 72) EMILIANI RIGATONI WITH EMERALD SAUCE

| Preparation Time: 10 minutes | Cooking Time: 20-30 minutes | Servings: 2 |
|---|---|---|

**Ingredients:**

- ✓ 260 g kale
- ✓ One clove of garlic.
- ✓ 4 oz of olive oil.
- ✓ Twelve ounces of rigatoni.
- ✓ One and a half tbsp of freshly grated parmesan.
- ✓ ¼ tsp of black pepper.

**Directions:**

- ❖ Remove the stalk from kale leaves.
- ❖ Blanch the leaves into the boiling water along with garlic clove for draining up to 3 min.
- ❖ Take a food processor and put kale & garlic into it & blend to puree. Pour the olive oil in it & process until it becomes smooth.
- ❖ Cook rigatoni according to the direction given in the package.
- ❖ Place pasta into a bowl & add the sauce to it. Mix it well.
- ❖ Divide this into the bowls for serving and add parmesan cheese over it. Top it with black pepper.

**Nutrition:** Calories: 414, kcal Fat: 30 g Protein: 7g Carbs: 30g Fiber: 2g

## 73) KOREAN-STYLE MUSHROOM BIBIMBAP

| Preparation Time: 25 minutes | Cooking Time: 25-30 minutes | Servings: 4 |
|---|---|---|

**Ingredients:**

- ✓ BIBIMBAP
- ✓ 1 cup of Japanese rice
- ✓ One and a half tbsp of olive oil
- ✓ Four ounces of thin-sliced oyster mushrooms.
- ✓ 4 ounces of sliced cremini mushrooms
- ✓ Half cucumber peeled and sliced.
- ✓ Coating Spray thin.
- ✓ Four eggs
- ✓ one grated garlic clove.
- ✓ 1 cup spinach.
- ✓ Two tsp of Japanese seaweed.
- ✓ Sriracha sauce (optional)
- ✓ Gochujang paste (optional)
- ✓ 1/4 cup of sprouts, any type (optional)
- ✓ DRESSING
- ✓ 1 ½ tbsp of Japanese low sodium soy sauce.
- ✓ 1 tbsp of sesame oil
- ✓ 1 tbsp of rice vinegar
- ✓ 2 tsp of honey

**Directions:**

- ❖ Cook the rice according to the direction given by the package
- ❖ Heat 1 tbsp of olive oil on moderate heat.
- ❖ Sauté mushrooms for 5 min.
- ❖ Lower the heat. Add additional half tbsp olive oil seven cooks for more than 10 minutes.
- ❖ Combine all ingredients for the dressing.
- ❖ Pour 1/2 of dressing over cucumbers in a small bowl.
- ❖ Heat one separate small pan over moderate heat with cooking spray. Now cook the egg according to your wish.
- ❖ Add the garlic & the spinach into mushrooms. Sauté for 2 min till the spinach wilts. Continue stirring
- ❖ pour remaining dressing on the cooked vegetables & mix well.
- ❖ Divide the rice into four individual serving bowls. Arrange the mushroom mixture, cucumber & sprouts on the rice.
- ❖ Top every bowl with one cooked egg.
- ❖ Garnish using Japanese seasoning.
- ❖ Add a dollop of sriracha sauce for additional flavor. Top with the sprouts.

**Nutrition:** Calories:350 kcal Fat:13 g Protein: 10 g Carbs: 47g Fiber: 3g

## 74) MOROCCAN BULGUR WHEAT SALAD WITH CHICKEN IN POMEGRANATE MOLASSES

| Preparation Time: 15 minutes | Cooking Time: 10 minutes | Servings: 4 |
|---|---|---|

**Ingredients:**

- ✓ One small red onion, thinly sliced
- ✓ 100 g feta, crumbled
- ✓ 2 tbsp mint, thinly shredded
- ✓ 2 x 250 g bulgur wheat, chickpeas, and quinoa
- ✓ 2½ tbsp pomegranate molasses
- ✓ 40 g chopped pistachios
- ✓ 460 g chicken breasts
- ✓ 1 tsp sunflower oil
- ✓ 50 g pomegranate seeds

**Directions:**

- ❖ Preheat oven to 400 F. Take an ovenproof frying pan and heat the oil in it over medium heat. Season the chicken breasts with spices and fry them for 2-3 minutes on both sides in the pan.
- ❖ Retract the pan off the fire and sprinkle 1½ tbsp of pomegranate molasses with the chicken. Transfer to oven and cook until the mixture is fully cooked, for about 8 minutes or. Take out of the oven and allow for a couple of minutes to rest.
- ❖ Meanwhile, following the directions on the box, cook the grains. Mix with the feta, mint, red onion, and pomegranate seeds.
- ❖ Divide the mixture of grains into four serving plates. Cut the chicken and the leftover pomegranate molasses, pass to the dishes, and drizzle. To toast, cover with pistachios.

**Nutrition:** Calories: 198 kcal Fat: 17 g Protein: 44.5 g Carbs: 7.8 g Fiber: 7.8 g

## 75) EASY BROCCOLI AND CAPSICUM PASTA SALAD

| Preparation Time: 8 hours 30 minutes | Cooking Time: 20 minutes | Servings: 6 |
|---|---|---|

| | | |
|---|---|---|
| ✓ 350 g broccoli florets<br>✓ 280 g radiator pasta<br>✓ 175 g yellow or red grape tomatoes<br>✓ One yellow zucchini, thinly sliced<br>✓ One red onion, chopped | ✓ One large sliced red capsicum<br>✓ Dressing<br>✓ 20 g chopped fresh parsley<br>✓ 80 ml of olive oil<br>✓ 150 ml cider vinegar<br>✓ 2 tbsp chopped fresh dill<br>✓ pepper to taste | ❖ 1. Put out a big iced water cup. Over a high flame, put a big saucepan of water to a boil. In a broad metal sieve, placed the broccoli, red capsicum, onion, and zucchini. Immerse and blanch in the pool for about 2 minutes or before the shades brighten. Drain and lift, then dive into the cold sea.<br>❖ 2. In a saucepan of boiling water, cook the pasta according to the package directions. Drain and position in a large bowl for serving. Wash the vegetables and add them and also the tomatoes to the pasta.<br>❖ 3. lace the vinegar, oil, dill, parsley, and pepper in a container with a tight-fitting lid to make the seasoning, and shake until fully mixed. To coat, pour on the salad and toss gently. For at least 8 hours or overnight, cover and refrigerate. Until serving, toss again. |

## 76) ITALIAN SESAME SALAD DRESSING

| Preparation Time: 3 minutes | Cooking Time: 3 minutes | Servings: 1 |
|---|---|---|

| | | |
|---|---|---|
| ✓ 1/4 cup olive oil<br>✓ 1/4 cup soy sauce<br>✓ 1/4 cup white vinegar | ✓ 1 1/2 tbsp honey<br>✓ 2 tbsp toasted sesame oil | **Directions:**<br>❖ 1. In a container, put the ingredients and shake until the sugar dissolves. Change saltiness with the salt and sugar with sweetness to taste.<br>❖ 2. Leave it in the fridge for up to 3 weeks (to be safe). Take to room temperature and shake well before use.<br>❖ 3.For 3 to 4 cups of chopped cabbage or leafy greens, the side salad for four persons, a single serving dish is enough. |

## 77) MEXICAN-STYLE TORTILLA SOUP

| | Cooking Time: 40 Minutes | Servings: 4 |
|---|---|---|

| | | |
|---|---|---|
| ✓ 1-pound chicken breasts, boneless and skinless<br>✓ 1 can (15 ounces whole peeled tomatoes<br>✓ 1 can (10 ounces red enchilada sauce<br>✓ 1 and 1/2 tsp minced garlic<br>✓ 1 yellow onion, diced<br>✓ 1 can (4 ounces fire-roasted diced green chile<br>✓ 1 can (15 ounces black beans, drained and rinsed | ✓ 1 can (15 ounces fire-roasted corn, undrained<br>✓ 1 container (32 ounces chicken stock or broth<br>✓ 1 tsp ground cumin<br>✓ 2 tsp chili powder<br>✓ 3/4 tsp paprika<br>✓ 1 bay leaf<br>✓ Salt and freshly cracked pepper, to taste<br>✓ 1 tbsp chopped cilantro<br>✓ Tortilla strips, Freshly squeezed lime juice, freshly grated cheddar cheese, | **Directions:**<br>❖ Set your Instant Pot on Sauté mode.<br>❖ Toss olive oil, onion and garlic into the insert of the Instant Pot.<br>❖ Sauté for 4 minutes then add chicken and remaining ingredients.<br>❖ Mix well gently then seal and lock the lid.<br>❖ Select Manual mode for 7 minutes at high pressure.<br>❖ Once done, release the pressure completely then remove the lid.<br>❖ Adjust seasoning as needed.<br>❖ Garnish with desired toppings.<br>❖ Enjoy. |

**Nutrition:** Calories: 390;Carbohydrate: 5.6g;Protein: 29.5g;Fat: 26.5g;Sugar: 2.1g;Sodium: 620mg

## 78) ITALIAN CHICKEN SOUP

| | Cooking Time: 35 Minutes | Servings: 6 |
|---|---|---|

**Ingredients:**

- ✓ 1 tbsp olive oil
- ✓ 1 1/2 cups peeled and diced carrots
- ✓ 1 1/2 cup diced celery
- ✓ 1 cup chopped yellow onion
- ✓ 3 tbsp minced garlic
- ✓ 8 cups low-sodium chicken broth
- ✓ 2 tsp minced fresh thyme
- ✓ 2 tsp minced fresh rosemary
- ✓ 1 bay leaf
- ✓ salt and freshly ground black pepper
- ✓ 2 1/2 lbs. bone-in, skin-on chicken thighs, skinned
- ✓ 3 cups wide egg noodles, such as American beauty
- ✓ 1 tbsp fresh lemon juice
- ✓ 1/4 cup chopped fresh parsley

**Directions:**

- ❖ Preheat olive oil in the insert of the Instant Pot on Sauté mode.
- ❖ Add onion, celery, and carrots and sauté them for minutes.
- ❖ Stir in garlic and sauté for 1 minute.
- ❖ Add bay leaf, thyme, broth, rosemary, salt, and pepper.
- ❖ Seal and secure the Instant Pot lid and select Manual mode for 10 minutes at high pressure.
- ❖ Once done, release the pressure completely then remove the lid.
- ❖ Add noodles to the insert and switch the Instant Pot to sauté mode.
- ❖ Cook the soup for 6 minutes until noodles are all done.
- ❖ Remove the chicken and shred it using a fork.
- ❖ Return the chicken to the soup then add lemon juice and parsley.
- ❖ Enjoy.

## 79) SPECIAL TURKEY ARUGULA SALAD

| | Cooking Time: 5 Minutes | Servings: 2 |
|---|---|---|

**Ingredients:**

- ✓ 4 oz turkey breast meat, diced into small pieces
- ✓ 3.5 oz arugula leaves
- ✓ 10 raspberries
- ✓ Juice from ½ a lime
- ✓ 2 tbsp extra virgin olive oil

**Directions:**

- ❖ Mix together the turkey with the rest of the ingredients in a large bowl until well combined.
- ❖ Dish out in a glass bowl and serve immediately.

## 80) SPECIAL CHEESY BROCCOLI SOUP

| | Cooking Time: 30 Minutes | Servings: 4 |
|---|---|---|

**Ingredients:**

- ✓ ½ cup heavy whipping cream
- ✓ 1 cup broccoli
- ✓ 1 cup cheddar cheese
- ✓ Salt, to taste
- ✓ 1½ cups chicken broth

**Directions:**

- ❖ Heat chicken broth in a large pot and add broccoli.
- ❖ Bring to a boil and stir in the rest of the ingredients.
- ❖ Allow the soup to simmer on low heat for about 20 minutes.
- ❖ Ladle out into a bowl and serve hot.

**Nutrition:** Calories: 188;Carbs: 2.6g;Fats: 15g;Proteins: 9.8g;Sodium: 514mg;Sugar: 0.8g

## 81) DELICIOUS RICH POTATO SOUP

| | Cooking Time: 30 Minutes | Servings: 4 |
|---|---|---|

**Ingredients:**

- ✓ 1 tbsp butter
- ✓ 1 medium onion, diced
- ✓ 3 cloves garlic, minced
- ✓ 3 cups chicken broth
- ✓ 1 can/box cream of chicken soup
- ✓ 7-8 medium-sized russet potatoes, peeled and chopped
- ✓ 1 1/2 tsp salt
- ✓ Black pepper to taste
- ✓ 1 cup milk
- ✓ 1 tbsp flour
- ✓ 2 cups shredded cheddar cheese
- ✓ Garnish:
- ✓ 5-6 slices bacon, chopped
- ✓ Sliced green onions
- ✓ Shredded cheddar cheese

**Directions:**

- ❖ Heat butter in the insert of the Instant Pot on sauté mode.
- ❖ Add onions and sauté for 4 minutes until soft.
- ❖ Stir in garlic and sauté it for 1 minute.
- ❖ Add potatoes, cream of chicken, broth, salt, and pepper to the insert.
- ❖ Mix well then seal and lock the lid.
- ❖ Cook this mixture for 10 minutes at Manual Mode with high pressure.
- ❖ Meanwhile, mix flour with milk in a bowl and set it aside.
- ❖ Once the instant pot beeps, release the pressure completely.
- ❖ Remove the Instant Pot lid and switch the instant pot to Sauté mode.
- ❖ Pour in flour slurry and stir cook the mixture for 5 minutes until it thickens.
- ❖ Add 2 cups of cheddar cheese and let it melt.
- ❖ Garnish it as desired.
- ❖ Serve.

**Nutrition:** Calories: 784;Carbohydrate: 54.8g;Protein: 34g;Fat: 46.5g;Sugar: 7.5g;Sodium: 849mg

## 82) ITALIAN STYLE LENTIL SOUP

| | Cooking Time: 20 Minutes | Servings: 4 |
|---|---|---|

**Ingredients:**

- ✓ 1 tbsp olive oil
- ✓ 1/2 cup red lentils
- ✓ 1 medium yellow or red onion
- ✓ 2 garlic cloves, chopped
- ✓ 1/2 tsp ground cumin
- ✓ 1/2 tsp ground coriander
- ✓ 1/2 tsp ground sumac
- ✓ 1/2 tsp red chili flakes
- ✓ 1/2 tsp dried parsley
- ✓ 3/4 tsp dried mint flakes
- ✓ pinch of sugar
- ✓ 2.5 cups water
- ✓ salt, to taste
- ✓ black pepper, to taste
- ✓ juice of 1/2 lime
- ✓ parsley or cilantro, to garnish

**Directions:**

- ❖ Preheat oil in the insert of your Instant Pot on Sauté mode.
- ❖ Add onion and sauté until it turns golden brown.
- ❖ Toss in the garlic, parsley sugar, mint flakes, red chili flakes, sumac, coriander, and cumin.
- ❖ Stir cook this mixture for 2 minutes.
- ❖ Add water, lentils, salt, and pepper. Stir gently.
- ❖ Seal and lock the Instant Pot lid and select Manual mode for 8 minutes at high pressure.
- ❖ Once done, release the pressure completely then remove the lid.
- ❖ Stir well then add lime juice.
- ❖ Serve warm.

**Nutrition:** Calories: 525;Carbohydrate: 59.8g;Protein: 30.1g;Fat: 19.3g;Sugar: 17.3g;Sodium: 897mg

## 83) SPECIAL BUTTERNUT SQUASH SOUP

| | Cooking Time: 40 Minutes | Servings: 4 |
|---|---|---|

**Ingredients:**

- ✓ 1 tbsp olive oil
- ✓ 1 medium yellow onion chopped
- ✓ 1 large carrot chopped
- ✓ 1 celery rib chopped
- ✓ 3 cloves of garlic minced
- ✓ 2 lbs. butternut squash, peeled chopped
- ✓ 2 cups vegetable broth
- ✓ 1 green apple peeled, cored, and chopped
- ✓ 1/4 tsp ground cinnamon
- ✓ 1 sprig fresh thyme
- ✓ 1 sprig fresh rosemary
- ✓ 1 tsp kosher salt
- ✓ 1/2 tsp black pepper
- ✓ Pinch of nutmeg optional

**Directions:**

- ❖ Preheat olive oil in the insert of the Instant Pot on Sauté mode.
- ❖ Add celery, carrots, and garlic, sauté for 5 minutes.
- ❖ Stir in squash, broth, cinnamon, apple nutmeg, rosemary, thyme, salt, and pepper.
- ❖ Mix well gently then seal and secure the lid.
- ❖ Select Manual mode to cook for 10 minutes at high pressure.
- ❖ Once done, release the pressure completely then remove the lid.
- ❖ Puree the soup using an immersion blender.
- ❖ Serve warm.

## 84) LOVELY CREAMY CILANTRO AND LIME SALAD

| | Cooking Time: 10 Minutes | Servings: 2 |
|---|---|---|

**Ingredients:**

- ✓ ¾ avocado
- ✓ 1 lime, juiced
- ✓ 1/8 cup water
- ✓ Cilantro, to garnish
- ✓ 6 oz coleslaw, bagged
- ✓ 1/8 cup cilantro leaves
- ✓ 1 garlic clove
- ✓ ¼ tsp salt

**Directions:**

- ❖ Put garlic and cilantro in a food processor and process until chopped.
- ❖ Add lime juice, avocado and water and pulse until creamy.
- ❖ Put coleslaw in a large bowl and stir in the avocado mixture.
- ❖ Refrigerate for a few hours before serving.

## 85) CLASSIC SNAP PEA SALAD

| | Cooking Time: 15 Minutes | Servings: 2 |
|---|---|---|

- ✓ 1/8 cup lemon juice
- ✓ ½ clove garlic, crushed
- ✓ 4 ounces cauliflower riced
- ✓ 1/8 cup olive oil
- ✓ ¼ tsp coarse grain Dijon mustard
- ✓ ½ tsp granulated stevia
- ✓ ¼ cup sugar snap peas, ends removed and each pod cut into three pieces
- ✓ 1/8 cup chives
- ✓ 1/8 cup red onions, minced
- ✓ Sea salt and black pepper, to taste
- ✓ ¼ cup almonds, sliced

**Directions:**

- ❖ Pour water in a pot fitted with a steamer basket and bring water to a boil.
- ❖ Place riced cauliflower in the steamer basket and season with sea salt.
- ❖ Cover the pot and steam for about 10 minutes until tender.
- ❖ Drain the cauliflower and dish out in a bowl to refrigerate for about 1 hour.
- ❖ Meanwhile, make a dressing by mixing olive oil, lemon juice, garlic, mustard, stevia, salt and black pepper in a bowl.
- ❖ Mix together chilled cauliflower, peas, chives, almonds and red onions in another bowl.
- ❖ Pour the dressing over this mixture and serve.

**Nutrition:** Calories: 203;Carbs: 7.6g;Fats: 18g;Proteins: 4.2g;Sodium: 28mg;Sugar: 2.9g

## 86) SPINACH AND BACON SALAD

| | Cooking Time: 15 Minutes | Servings: 4 |
|---|---|---|

| Ingredients: | ✓ 8 pieces thick bacon, cooked and sliced | Directions: |
|---|---|---|
| ✓ 2 eggs, boiled, halved, and sliced | ✓ ½ cup plain mayonnaise | ❖ Mix together the mayonnaise and spinach in a large bowl. |
| ✓ 10 oz. organic baby spinach, rinsed, and dried | ✓ ½ medium red onion, thinly sliced | ❖ Stir in the rest of the ingredients and combine well. |
| | | ❖ Dish out in a glass bowl and serve well. |

Nutrition: Calories: 373;Carbs: ;Fats: 34.5g;Proteins: 11g;Sodium: 707mg;Sugar: 1.1g

## 87) TYPICAL BEEF STROGANOFF SOUP

| | Cooking Time: 35 Minutes | Servings: 6 |
|---|---|---|

| Ingredients: | ✓ salt and pepper to taste | Directions: |
|---|---|---|
| ✓ 1.5 pounds stew meat | ✓ 1/2 cup sour cream | ❖ Add meat, 5 cups broth, Italian seasoning, Worcestershire sauce, garlic powder, salt, pepper, and onion powder to the insert of the Instant Pot. |
| ✓ 6 cups beef broth | ✓ 8 ounces mushrooms, sliced | ❖ Secure and seal the Instant Pot lid then select Manual mode for 1 hour at high pressure. |
| ✓ 4 tbsp Worcestershire sauce | ✓ 8 ounces short noodles, cooked | ❖ Once done, release the pressure completely then remove the lid. |
| ✓ 1/2 tsp Italian seasoning blend | ✓ 1/3 cup cold water | ❖ Set the Instant pot on Soup mode and add sour cream along with 1 cup broth. |
| ✓ 1 1/2 tsp onion powder | ✓ 1/4 cup corn starch | ❖ Mix well then add mushrooms and mix well. |
| ✓ 2 tsp garlic powder | | ❖ Whisk corn-starch with water and pour this mixture into the pot. |
| | | ❖ Cook this mixture until it thickens then add noodles, salt, and pepper. |
| | | ❖ Garnish with cheese parsley, black pepper. |
| | | ❖ Enjoy. |

## 88) EGG, AVOCADO WITH TOMATO SALAD

| | Cooking Time: 40 Minutes | Servings: 4 |
|---|---|---|

| Ingredients: | ✓ 1 medium-sized tomato, chopped into chunks | Directions: |
|---|---|---|
| ✓ 2 boiled eggs, chopped into chunks | ✓ Salt and black pepper, to taste | ❖ Mix together all the ingredients in a large bowl until well combined. |
| ✓ 1 ripe avocado, chopped into chunks | ✓ 1 lemon wedge, juiced | ❖ Dish out in a glass bowl and serve immediately. |

Nutrition: Calories: 140;Carbs: 5.9g;Fats: 12.1g;Proteins: 4g;Sodium: mg;Sugar: 1.3g

## 89) SPECIAL LOW-CARB CREAMY BUTTERNUT SQUASH SOUP

| | **Cooking Time:** 1 Hour 10 Minutes | **Servings: 8** |
|---|---|---|

| Ingredients | Ingredients | Directions |
|---|---|---|
| ✓ 2 tbsp avocado oil, divided<br>✓ 2 pounds butternut squash, cut in half length-wise and seeds removed | ✓ Sea salt and black pepper, to taste<br>✓ 1 (13.5-oz can coconut milk<br>✓ 4 cups chicken bone broth | ❖ Preheat the oven to 400 degrees F and grease a baking sheet.<br>❖ Arrange the butternut squash halves with open side up on the baking sheet.<br>❖ Drizzle with half of the avocado oil and season with sea salt and black pepper.<br>❖ Flip over and transfer into the oven.<br>❖ Roast the butternut squash for about minutes.<br>❖ Heat the remaining avocado oil over medium heat in a large pot and add the broth and coconut milk.<br>❖ Let it simmer for about 20 minutes and scoop the squash out of the shells to transfer into the soup.<br>❖ Puree this mixture in an immersion blender until smooth and serve immediately. |

## 90) Easy Skinny slow cooker kale and turkey meatball soup

| **Preparation Time:** 15 minutes | **Cooking Time:** 240 minutes | **Servings: 4** |
|---|---|---|

| Ingredients | Ingredients | Directions: |
|---|---|---|
| ✓ ¼ cup milk<br>✓ 1 lb lean turkey<br>✓ Two slices of bread<br>✓ One chopped shallot<br>✓ ½ tsp grated nutmeg<br>✓ Two chopped garlic cloves<br>✓ 1 tsp oregano<br>✓ Kosher salt to taste<br>✓ 1/4 tsp red pepper flakes | ✓ Black pepper to taste<br>✓ 2 tbsp chopped parsley<br>✓ ½ cup grated Parmigiano-Reggiano<br>✓ One egg<br>✓ 8 cups chicken broth<br>✓ 1 tbsp olive oil<br>✓ 15 oz white beans<br>✓ ½ chopped onion<br>✓ Two sliced carrots<br>✓ 4 cups kale | ❖ Soak pieces of bread in milk in a bowl followed by the addition of nutmeg, flakes, cheese, turkey, parsley, shallot, oregano, salt, egg, garlic, and pepper.<br>❖ Mix well using hands. Make meatballs out of the turkey mixture.<br>❖ Fry meatballs in heat olive oil in a skillet over a high flame. Keep the fried meatballs aside for a few minutes.<br>❖ Place beans, onions, carrot, kale, and broth in a slow cooker, followed by adding meatballs in broth.<br>❖ Cover the cooker and cook for four hours.<br>❖ Garnish with grated cheese, parsley, and flakes and serve. |

**Nutrition:** Calories: 297 kcal Fat: 10 g Protein: 21 g Carbs: 27 g Fiber: 2 g

## 91) SPECIAL SANDWICH WITH CHICKEN CAPRESE

| **Preparation Time:** 10 minutes | **Cooking Time:** 6 minutes | **Servings: 4** |
|---|---|---|

| Ingredients | Ingredients | Directions |
|---|---|---|
| ✓ 4 tbsp olive oil<br>✓ 1 tbsp lemon juice<br>✓ ¼ cup basil leaves<br>✓ 1 tsp minced parsley<br>✓ Kosher salt to taste<br>✓ Two boneless chicken breasts | ✓ Black pepper to taste<br>✓ 10 oz sliced sourdough bread<br>✓ Eleven Campari tomatoes<br>✓ 8 oz sliced mozzarella cheese<br>✓ Balsamic vinegar as required | ❖ Add chicken pieces, olive oil, lemon juice, salt, parsley, and pepper in a bowl. Toss well to coat chicken evenly. Set aside.<br>❖ Grill the chicken on a preheated grill on a medium flame for six minutes from both sides.<br>❖ Toast the bread drizzled with olive oil.<br>❖ Sliced the bread into three pieces.<br>❖ Place chicken pieces, cheese, and tomato slices over each slice of bread.<br>❖ Sprinkle vinegar, oil, salt, basil, and pepper over the bread slices and serve. |

**Nutrition:** Calories: 612.73 kcal Fat: 32.06 g Protein: 34.4 g Carbs: 46.88 g Fiber: 2.25 g

## 92) AUTHENTIC MINESTRONE

| Preparation Time: 15 minutes | Cooking Time: 30 minutes | Servings: 6 |
|---|---|---|

**Ingredients:**

- ✓ 2 tbsp olive oil
- ✓ 1/3 cup shredded parmesan cheese
- ✓ Four chopped garlic cloves
- ✓ One chopped onion
- ✓ Two chopped celery stalks
- ✓ 1/3 lb green beans
- ✓ One diced carrot
- ✓ 1 tsp oregano
- ✓ Salt to taste
- ✓ 1 tsp basil
- ✓ Black pepper to taste
- ✓ 14 oz crushed tomatoes
- ✓ 28 oz diced tomatoes
- ✓ 6 cups chicken stock
- ✓ 1 cup elbow pasta
- ✓ 15 oz beans
- ✓ 2 tbsp chopped basil

**Directions:**

- ❖ Sauté onions in heated olive oil over medium flame for five minutes.
- ❖ Stir in garlic and cook for half a minute.
- ❖ Mix carrot and celery and cook for five more minutes with occasional stirring.
- ❖ Add oregano, beans, salt, basil, and black pepper and cook for another three minutes with constant stirring.
- ❖ Pour broth followed by the addition of tomatoes and let it boil.
- ❖ Lower the flame to low and let it simmer for ten minutes.
- ❖ Add pasta and kidney beans and cook for another ten minutes. Mix salt and serve after garnishing with cheese and bail.

**Nutrition:** Calories: 260 kcal Fat: 8 g Protein: 15 g Carbs: 37 g Fiber: 10 g

## 93) SPECIAL FRUIT SALAD WITH MINT AND ORANGE BLOSSOM WATER

| | Cooking Time: 10 Minutes | Servings: 5 |
|---|---|---|

**Ingredients:**

- ✓ 3 cups cantaloupe, cut into 1-inch cubes
- ✓ 2 cups hulled and halved strawberries
- ✓ ½ tsp orange blossom water
- ✓ 2 tbsp chopped fresh mint

**Directions:**

- ❖ In a large bowl, toss all the ingredients together.
- ❖ Place 1 cup of fruit salad in each of 5 containers.
- ❖ STORAGE: Store covered containers in the refrigerator for up to 5 days.

**Nutrition:** Total calories: 52; Total fat: 1g; Saturated fat: <1g; Sodium: 10mg; Carbohydrates: 12g; Fiber: 2g; Protein: 1g

## 94) ROASTED BROCCOLI WITH RED ONIONS AND POMEGRANATE SEEDS

| | Cooking Time: 20 Minutes | Servings: 5 |
|---|---|---|

**Ingredients:**

- ✓ 1 (12-ounce) package broccoli florets (about 6 cups)
- ✓ 1 small red onion, thinly sliced
- ✓ 2 tbsp olive oil
- ✓ ¼ tsp kosher salt
- ✓ 1 (5.3-ounce) container pomegranate seeds (1 cup)

**Directions:**

- ❖ Preheat the oven to 425°F and line 2 sheet pans with silicone baking mats or parchment paper.
- ❖ Place the broccoli and onion on the sheet pans and toss with the oil and salt. Place the pans in the oven and roast for minutes.
- ❖ After removing the pans from the oven, cool the veggies, then toss with the pomegranate seeds.
- ❖ Place 1 cup of veggies in each of 5 containers.
- ❖ STORAGE: Store covered containers in the refrigerator for up to days.

## 95) DELICIOUS CHERMOULA SAUCE

| | **Cooking Time:** 10 Minutes | **Servings: 1 Cup** |
|---|---|---|

**Ingredients:**

- ✓ 1 cup packed parsley leaves
- ✓ 1 cup cilantro leaves
- ✓ ½ cup mint leaves
- ✓ 1 tsp chopped garlic
- ✓ ½ tsp ground cumin
- ✓ ½ tsp ground coriander
- ✓ ½ tsp smoked paprika
- ✓ ⅛ tsp cayenne pepper
- ✓ ⅛ tsp kosher salt
- ✓ 3 tbsp freshly squeezed lemon juice
- ✓ 3 tbsp water
- ✓ ½ cup extra-virgin olive oil

**Directions:**

- ❖ Place all the ingredients in a blender or food processor and blend until smooth.
- ❖ Pour the chermoula into a container and refrigerate.
- ❖ STORAGE: Store the covered container in the refrigerator for up to 5 days.

## 96) DEVILED EGG PESTO WITH SUN-DRIED TOMATOES

| | **Cooking Time:** 15 Minutes | **Servings: 5** |
|---|---|---|

**Ingredients:**

- ✓ 5 large eggs
- ✓ 3 tbsp prepared pesto
- ✓ ¼ tsp white vinegar
- ✓ 2 tbsp low-fat (2%) plain Greek yogurt
- ✓ 5 tsp sliced sun-dried tomatoes

- ❖ Place the eggs in a saucepan and cover with water. Bring the water to a boil. As soon as the water starts to boil, place a lid on the pan and turn the heat off. Set a timer for minutes.
- ❖ When the timer goes off, drain the hot water and run cold water over the eggs to cool.
- ❖ Peel the eggs, slice in half vertically, and scoop out the yolks. Place the yolks in a medium mixing bowl and add the pesto, vinegar, and yogurt. Mix well, until creamy.
- ❖ Scoop about 1 tbsp of the pesto-yolk mixture into each egg half. Top each with ½ tsp of sun-dried tomatoes.
- ❖ Place 2 stuffed egg halves in each of separate containers.
- ❖ STORAGE: Store covered containers in the refrigerator for up to 5 days.

## 97) WHITE BEAN WITH MUSHROOM DIP

| | **Cooking Time:** 8 Minutes | **Servings: 3 Cups** |
|---|---|---|

- ✓
- ✓ 2 tsp olive oil, plus 2 tbsp
- ✓ 8 ounces button or cremini mushrooms, sliced
- ✓ 1 tsp chopped garlic
- ✓ 1 tbsp fresh thyme leaves
- ✓ 2 (15.5-ounce) cans cannellini beans, drained and rinsed
- ✓ 2 tbsp plus 1 tsp freshly squeezed lemon juice
- ✓ ½ tsp kosher salt

- ❖ Heat 2 tsp of oil in a -inch skillet over medium-high heat. Once the oil is shimmering, add the mushrooms and sauté for 6 minutes. Add the garlic and thyme and continue cooking for 2 minutes.
- ❖ While the mushrooms are cooking, place the beans and lemon juice, the remaining tbsp of oil, and the salt in the bowl of a food processor. Add the mushrooms as soon as they are done cooking and blend everything until smooth. Scrape down the sides of the bowl if necessary and continue to process until smooth.
- ❖ Taste and adjust the seasoning with lemon juice or salt if needed.
- ❖ Scoop the dip into a container and refrigerate.
- ❖ STORAGE: Store the covered container in the refrigerator for up to days. Dip can be frozen for up to 3 months.

## 98) SPICY SAUTÉED CABBAGE IN NORTH AFRICAN STYLE

| | Cooking Time: 10 Minutes | Servings: 4 |
|---|---|---|

| Ingredients: | ✓ ½ tsp caraway seeds | Directions: |
|---|---|---|
| ✓ 2 tsp olive oil<br>✓ 1 small head green cabbage (about 1½ to 2 pounds), cored and thinly sliced<br>✓ 1 tsp ground coriander<br>✓ 1 tsp garlic powder | ✓ ½ tsp ground cumin<br>✓ ¼ tsp kosher salt<br>✓ Pinch red chili flakes (optional—if you don't like heat, omit it)<br>✓ 1 tsp freshly squeezed lemon juice | ❖ Heat the oil in a -inch skillet over medium-high heat. Once the oil is hot, add the cabbage and cook down for 3 minutes. Add the coriander, garlic powder, caraway seeds, cumin, salt, and chili flakes (if using) and stir to combine. Continue cooking the cabbage for about 7 more minutes.<br>❖ Stir in the lemon juice and cool.<br>❖ Place 1 heaping cup of cabbage in each of 4 containers.<br>❖ STORAGE: Store covered containers in the refrigerator for up to 5 days. |

## 99) FLAX, BLUEBERRY, AND SUNFLOWER BUTTER BITES

| | Cooking Time: 10 Minutes | Servings: 6 |
|---|---|---|

| ✓ ½ cup unsweetened sunflower butter, preferably unsalted<br>✓ ⅓ cup dried blueberries<br>✓ 2 tbsp all-fruit blueberry preserves | ✓ Zest of 1 lemon<br>✓ 2 tbsp unsalted sunflower seeds<br>✓ ⅓ cup rolled oats<br>✓ ¼ cup ground flaxseed | ❖ Mix all the ingredients in a medium mixing bowl until well combined.<br>❖ Form 1balls, slightly smaller than a golf ball, from the mixture and place on a plate in the freezer for about 20 minutes to firm up.<br>❖ Place 2 bites in each of 6 containers and refrigerate.<br>❖ STORAGE: Store covered containers in the refrigerator for up to 5 days. Bites may also be stored in the freezer for up to 3 months. |

## 100) SPECIAL DIJON RED WINE VINAIGRETTE

| | Cooking Time: 5 Minutes | Servings: ½ Cup |
|---|---|---|

| ✓ 2 tsp Dijon mustard<br>✓ 3 tbsp red wine vinegar<br>✓ 1 tbsp water | ✓ ¼ tsp dried oregano<br>✓ ¼ tsp chopped garlic<br>✓ ⅛ tsp kosher salt<br>✓ ¼ cup olive oil | ❖ Place the mustard, vinegar, water, oregano, garlic, and salt in a small bowl and whisk to combine.<br>❖ Whisk in the oil, pouring it into the mustard-vinegar mixture in a thin steam.<br>❖ Pour the vinaigrette into a container and refrigerate.<br>❖ STORAGE: Store the covered container in the refrigerator for up to 2 weeks. Allow the vinaigrette to come to room temperature and shake before serving. |

## 101) DELICIOUS CREAMY KETO CUCUMBER SALAD

| | Cooking Time: 5 Minutes | Servings: 2 |
|---|---|---|

| ✓ 2 tbsp mayonnaise<br>✓ Salt and black pepper, to taste | ✓ 1 cucumber, sliced and quartered<br>✓ 2 tbsp lemon juice | ❖ Mix together the mayonnaise, cucumber slices, and lemon juice in a large bowl.<br>❖ Season with salt and black pepper and combine well.<br>❖ Dish out in a glass bowl and serve while it is cold. |

## 102) CABBAGE SOUP WITH SAUSAGE AND MUSHROOMS

| | Cooking Time: 1 Hour 10 Minutes | Servings: 6 |
|---|---|---|

**Ingredients:**

- ✓ 2 cups fresh kale, cut into bite sized pieces
- ✓ 6.5 ounces mushrooms, sliced
- ✓ 6 cups chicken bone broth
- ✓ 1 pound sausage, cooked and sliced
- ✓ Salt and black pepper, to taste

**Directions:**

- ❖ Heat chicken broth with two cans of water in a large pot and bring to a boil.
- ❖ Stir in the rest of the ingredients and allow the soup to simmer on low heat for about 1 hour.
- ❖ Dish out and serve hot.

**Nutrition:** Calories: 259;Carbs: ;Fats: 20g;Proteins: 14g;Sodium: 995mg;Sugar: 0.6g

## 103) CLASSIC MINESTRONE SOUP

| | Cooking Time: 25 Minutes | Servings: 6 |
|---|---|---|

- ✓ 2 tbsp olive oil
- ✓ 3 cloves garlic, minced
- ✓ 1 onion, diced
- ✓ 2 carrots, peeled and diced
- ✓ 2 stalks celery, diced
- ✓ 1 1/2 tsp dried basil
- ✓ 1 tsp dried oregano
- ✓ 1/2 tsp fennel seed
- ✓ 6 cups low sodium chicken broth
- ✓ 1 (28-ounce can diced tomatoes
- ✓ 1 (16-ounce can kidney beans, drained and rinsed
- ✓ 1 zucchini, chopped
- ✓ 1 (3-inch Parmesan rind
- ✓ 1 bay leaf
- ✓ 1 bunch kale leaves, chopped
- ✓ 2 tsp red wine vinegar
- ✓ Kosher salt and black pepper, to taste
- ✓ 1/3 cup freshly grated Parmesan
- ✓ 2 tbsp chopped fresh parsley leaves

- ❖ Preheat olive oil in the insert of the Instant Pot on Sauté mode.
- ❖ Add carrots, celery, and onion, sauté for 3 minutes.
- ❖ Stir in fennel seeds, oregano, and basil. Stir cook for 1 minute.
- ❖ Add stock, beans, tomatoes, parmesan, bay leaf, and zucchini.
- ❖ Secure and seal the Instant Pot lid then select Manual mode to cook for minutes at high pressure.
- ❖ Once done, release the pressure completely then remove the lid.
- ❖ Add kale and let it sit for 2 minutes in the hot soup.
- ❖ Stir in red wine, vinegar, pepper, and salt.
- ❖ Garnish with parsley and parmesan.
- ❖ Enjoy.

## 104) SPECIAL SALAD OF KOMBU SEAWEED

| | Cooking Time: 40 Minutes | Servings: 6 |
|---|---|---|

- ✓ 4 garlic cloves, crushed
- ✓ 1 pound fresh kombu seaweed, boiled and cut into strips
- ✓ 2 tbsp apple cider vinegar
- ✓ Salt, to taste
- ✓ 2 tbsp coconut aminos

- ❖ Mix together the kombu, garlic, apple cider vinegar, and coconut aminos in a large bowl.
- ❖ Season with salt and combine well.
- ❖ Dish out in a glass bowl and serve immediately.

## 105) TURKEY MEATBALL WITH DITALINI SOUP

| | Cooking Time: 40 Minutes | Servings: 4 |
|---|---|---|

| Ingredients | | Directions |
|---|---|---|
| ✓ meatballs:<br>✓ 1 pound 93% lean ground turkey<br>✓ 1/3 cup seasoned breadcrumbs<br>✓ 3 tbsp grated Pecorino Romano cheese<br>✓ 1 large egg, beaten<br>✓ 1 clove crushed garlic<br>✓ 1 tbsp fresh minced parsley<br>✓ 1/2 tsp kosher salt<br>✓ Soup:<br>✓ cooking spray<br>✓ 1 tsp olive oil<br>✓ 1/2 cup chopped onion<br>✓ 1/2 cup chopped celery | ✓ 1/2 cup chopped carrot<br>✓ 3 cloves minced garlic<br>✓ 1 can (28 ounces diced San Marzano tomatoes<br>✓ 4 cups reduced sodium chicken broth<br>✓ 4 torn basil leaves<br>✓ 2 bay leaves<br>✓ 1 cup ditalini pasta<br>✓ 1 cup zucchini, diced small<br>✓ Parmesan rind, optional<br>✓ Grated parmesan cheese, optional for serving | ❖ Thoroughly combine turkey with egg, garlic, parsley, salt, pecorino and breadcrumbs in a bowl.<br>❖ Make 30 equal sized meatballs out of this mixture.<br>❖ Preheat olive oil in the insert of the Instant Pot on Sauté mode.<br>❖ Sear the meatballs in the heated oil in batches, until brown.<br>❖ Set the meatballs aside in a plate.<br>❖ Add more oil to the insert of the Instant Pot.<br>❖ Stir in carrots, garlic, celery, and onion. Sauté for 4 minutes.<br>❖ Add basil, bay leaves, tomatoes, and Parmesan rind.<br>❖ Return the seared meatballs to the pot along with the broth.<br>❖ Secure and sear the Instant Pot lid and select Manual mode for 15 minutes at high pressure.<br>❖ Once done, release the pressure completely then remove the lid.<br>❖ Add zucchini and pasta, cook it for 4 minutes on Sauté mode.<br>❖ Garnish with cheese and basil.<br>❖ Serve. |

## 106) NICE COLD AVOCADO AND MINT SOUP

| | Cooking Time: 5 Minutes | Servings: 2 |
|---|---|---|

| Ingredients: | | Directions: |
|---|---|---|
| ✓ 1 cup coconut milk, chilled<br>✓ 1 medium ripe avocado<br>✓ 1 tbsp lime juice | ✓ Salt, to taste<br>✓ 20 fresh mint leaves | ❖ Put all the ingredients into an immersion blender and blend until a thick mixture is formed.<br>❖ Allow to cool in the fridge for about 10 minutes and serve chilled. |

## 107) CLASSIC SPLIT PEA SOUP

| | Cooking Time: 30 Minutes | Servings: 6 |
|---|---|---|

| Ingredients: | | Directions: |
|---|---|---|
| ✓ 3 tbsp butter<br>✓ 1 onion diced<br>✓ 2 ribs celery diced<br>✓ 2 carrots diced<br>✓ 6 oz. diced ham | ✓ 1 lb. dry split peas sorted and rinsed<br>✓ 6 cups chicken stock<br>✓ 2 bay leaves<br>✓ kosher salt and black pepper | ❖ Set your Instant Pot on Sauté mode and melt butter in it.<br>❖ Stir in celery, onion, carrots, salt, and pepper.<br>❖ Sauté them for 5 minutes then stir in split peas, ham bone, chicken stock, and bay leaves.<br>❖ Seal and lock the Instant Pot lid then select Manual mode for 15 minutes at high pressure.<br>❖ Once done, release the pressure completely then remove the lid.<br>❖ Remove the ham bone and separate meat from the bone.<br>❖ Shred or dice the meat and return it to the soup.<br>❖ Adjust seasoning as needed then serve warm.<br>❖ Enjoy. |

## 108) BAKED FILLET OF SOLE ITALIAN STYLE

| | | |
|---|---|---|
| **Cooking Time:** 15 Minutes | | **Servings:** 6 |

| Ingredients | Ingredients | Instructions |
|---|---|---|
| ✓ 1 lime or lemon, juice of<br>✓ 1/2 cup extra virgin olive oil<br>✓ 3 tbsp unsalted melted vegan butter<br>✓ 2 shallots, thinly sliced<br>✓ 3 garlic cloves, thinly-sliced<br>✓ 2 tbsp capers<br>✓ 1.5 lb Sole fillet, about 10–12 thin fillets | ✓ 4–6 green onions, top trimmed, halved lengthwise<br>✓ 1 lime or lemon, sliced (optional)<br>✓ 3/4 cup roughly chopped fresh dill for garnish<br>✓ 1 tsp seasoned salt, or to your taste<br>✓ 3/4 tsp ground black pepper<br>✓ 1 tsp ground cumin<br>✓ 1 tsp garlic powder | ❖ Preheat over to 375-degree F<br>❖ In a small bowl, whisk together olive oil, lime juice, and melted butter with a sprinkle of seasoned salt, stir in the garlic, shallots, and capers.<br>❖ In a separate small bowl, mix together the pepper, cumin, seasoned salt, and garlic powder, season the fish fillets each on both sides<br>❖ On a large baking pan or dish, arrange the fish fillets and cover with the buttery lime<br>❖ Arrange the green onion halves and lime slices on top. Bake in 375 degrees F for 10-15 minutes, do not overcook<br>❖ Remove the fish fillets from the oven. Allow the dish to cool completely<br>❖ Distribute among the containers, store for 2-3 days<br>❖ To Serve: Reheat in the microwave for 1-2 minutes or until heated through. Garnish with the chopped fresh dill. Serve with your favorite and a fresh salad<br>❖ Recipe Notes: If you can't get your hands on a sole fillet, cook this recipe with a different white fish. Just remember to change the baking time since it will be different. |

## 109) BAKED CHICKEN BREAST

| | | |
|---|---|---|
| **Cooking Time:** 50 Minutes | | **Servings:** 2 |

| Ingredients | Ingredients | Instructions |
|---|---|---|
| ✓ 2 skinless and boneless chicken breasts (about 8 ounces each)<br>✓ salt<br>✓ ground black pepper<br>✓ ¼ cup olive oil | ✓ ¼ cup freshly squeezed lemon juice<br>✓ 1 garlic clove, minced<br>✓ ½ tsp dried oregano<br>✓ ¼ tsp dried thyme | ❖ Preheat oven to a temperature of 400 degrees F.<br>❖ Season the chicken breasts carefully with salt and pepper on all sides.<br>❖ Place the chicken in a bowl.<br>❖ Take another bowl and add olive oil, lemon juice, oregano, garlic, and thyme. Mix well to make the marinade.<br>❖ Pour the marinade on top of chicken breasts and allow to marinate for 10 minutes. Set an oven rack about inches above the heat source.<br>❖ Place the chicken breasts into a baking pan and pour extra marinade on top. Bake for about 35-45 minutes until the center is no longer pink and the juices run clear. Move the baking dish to top rack and broil for about 5 minutes. Cool, spread over containers with some side dish and enjoy! |

## 110) LEMON FISH GRILL

| | | |
|---|---|---|
| **Cooking Time:** 15 Minutes | | **Servings:** 4 |

| Ingredients | Ingredients | Instructions |
|---|---|---|
| ✓ ¼ tsp sea salt<br>✓ 3 to 4 lemons<br>✓ ¼ tsp ground black pepper | ✓ 4 ounces any fish fillets, such as salmon or cod<br>✓ 1 tbsp olive oil | ❖ Ensure that the fish fillets are dry. If you know or feel they are a bit damp, take a paper towel and pat them dry.<br>❖ Leave the fish fillets on the counter for 10 minutes so they can stand at room temperature. Turn on your grill to medium-high heat or set the temperature to 400 degrees Fahrenheit. Using nonstick cooking spray, coat the grill so the fish won't stick. Take one lemon and cut it in half. Set one of the halves aside and cut the remaining half into ¼-inch thick slices.<br>❖ Now, take the other half of the lemon and squeeze at least 1 tbsp of juice out into a small bowl. Add oil into the small bowl and whisk the ingredients together. Brush the fish with the lemon and oil mixture. Make sure you get both sides of the fish.<br>❖ Arrange the lemon slices on the grill in the shape of the fish, it might take about 3 to 4 slices for one fish. Place the fish on top of the lemon slices and grill the ingredients together. If you don't have a lid for your grill, cover it with a different lid that will fit or use aluminum foil.<br>❖ When the fish is about half-way done, turn it over so the other side is laying on top of the lemon slices. You will know the fish is done when it starts to look flaky and separates easily, which you can check by gently pressing a fork onto the fish. |

## 111)   BAKED BEANS ITALIAN STYLE

| Cooking Time: 15 To 20 Minutes. | Servings: 6 |
|---|---|

| | | |
|---|---|---|
| ✓ ½ cup chopped onion<br>✓ ¼ cup red wine vinegar<br>✓ ¼ tbsp ground cinnamon<br>✓ 15 ounces or 2 cans of great northern beans, do not drain | ✓ 2 tsp extra virgin olive oil<br>✓ 12 ounces tomato paste, low sodium<br>✓ ½ cup water | ❖ Turn a burner to medium heat and add oil to a saucepan.<br>❖ Add the onion and cook for 4 to 5 minutes. Stir well.<br>❖ Combine the vinegar, tomato paste, cinnamon, and water. Mix until all the ingredients are well combined.<br>❖ Switch the heat to a low setting.<br>❖ Using a colander, drain one can of beans and pour into the pan.<br>❖ Open the second can of beans and pour all of it, including the liquid, into the saucepan and stir.<br>❖ Continue to cook the beans for 10 minutes while stirring frequently.<br>❖ Serve and enjoy! |

**Nutrition:** calories: 236, fats: 3 grams, carbohydrates: 42 grams, protein: 10 grams

## 112)   POMODORO TILAPIA

| Cooking Time: 15 Minutes | Servings: 4 |
|---|---|

| Ingredients: | | Directions: |
|---|---|---|
| ✓ 3 tbsp sun-dried tomatoes packed in oil, drained (juice/oil reserved) and chopped<br>✓ 1 tbsp capers, drained<br>✓ 2 pieces tilapia | ✓ 1 tbsp oil from sun-dried tomatoes<br>✓ 1 tbsp lemon juice<br>✓ 2 tbsp Kalamata olives, pitted and chopped | ❖ Preheat oven to 375 degrees F.<br>❖ Add sun-dried tomatoes, capers, and olives to a bowl; stir well and set aside.<br>❖ Place the tilapia fillets side by side on a baking sheet.<br>❖ Drizzle with oil and lemon juice.<br>❖ Bake for about 10-1minutes.<br>❖ Check the fish after 10 minutes to see if they are flakey.<br>❖ Once done, top the fish with tomato mixture. |

**Nutrition:** Calories: , Total Fat: 4.4 g, Saturated Fat: 0.8 g, Cholesterol: 28 mg, Sodium: 122 mg, Total Carbohydrate: 0.8 g, Dietary Fiber: 0.3 g, Total Sugars: 0.3 g, Protein: 10.7 g, Vitamin D: 0 mcg, Calcium: 16 mg, Iron: 1 mg, Potassium: 26 mg

## 113)   LENTIL SOUP WITH CHICKEN

| Cooking Time: 45 Minutes | Servings: 4 |
|---|---|

| Ingredients: | | Directions: |
|---|---|---|
| ✓ 1 pound dried lentils<br>✓ 12 ounces boneless chicken thigh meat<br>✓ 7 cups water<br>✓ 1 small onion, diced<br>✓ 2 scallions, chopped<br>✓ ¼ cup chopped cilantro | ✓ 3 cloves garlic<br>✓ 1 medium tomato, diced<br>✓ 1 tsp garlic powder<br>✓ 1 tsp cumin<br>✓ ¼ tsp oregano<br>✓ ½ tsp paprika<br>✓ ½ tsp kosher salt | ❖ Add all of the listed Ingredients: to your Instant Pot.<br>❖ Set your pot to SOUP mode and cook for 30 minutes.<br>❖ Allow the pressure to release naturally.<br>❖ Take the chicken out and shred.<br>❖ Place the chicken back in the pot and stir.<br>❖ Pour to the jars.<br>❖ Enjoy! |

## 114)  ASPARAGUS WRAPPED WITH BACON

| | | Cooking Time: 30 Minutes | Servings: 2 |
|---|---|---|---|

| | | |
|---|---|---|
| ✓ 1/3 cup heavy whipping cream<br>✓ 2 bacon slices, precooked | ✓ 4 small spears asparagus<br>✓ Salt, to taste<br>✓ 1 tbsp butter | ❖ Preheat the oven to 360 degrees F and grease a baking sheet with butter.<br>❖ Meanwhile, mix cream, asparagus and salt in a bowl.<br>❖ Wrap the asparagus in bacon slices and arrange them in the baking dish.<br>❖ Transfer the baking dish in the oven and bake for about 20 minutes. Remove from the oven and serve hot. Place the bacon wrapped asparagus in a dish and set aside to cool for meal prepping. Divide it in 2 containers and cover the lid. Refrigerate for about 2 days and reheat in the microwave before serving. |

## 115)  COOL ITALIAN-STYLE FISH

| | | Cooking Time: 30 Minutes | Servings: 8 |
|---|---|---|---|

| | | |
|---|---|---|
| ✓ 6 ounces halibut fillets<br>✓ 1 large tomato, chopped<br>✓ 1 onion, chopped<br>✓ 5 ounces kalamata olives, pitted | ✓ ¼ cup capers<br>✓ ¼ cup olive oil<br>✓ 1 tbsp lemon juice<br>✓ Salt and pepper as needed<br>✓ 1 tbsp Greek seasoning | ❖ Pre-heat your oven to 350-degree Fahrenheit<br>❖ Transfer the halibut fillets on a large aluminum foil Season with Greek seasoning<br>❖ Take a bowl and add tomato, onion, olives, olive oil, capers, pepper, lemon juice and salt<br>❖ Mix well and spoon the tomato mix over the halibut Seal the edges and fold to make a packet Place the packet on a baking sheet and bake in your oven for 30-40 minutes Serve once the fish flakes off and enjoy!<br>❖ Meal Prep/Storage Options: Store in airtight containers in your fridge for 1-2 days. |

## 116)  FANCY LUNCHEON SALAD

| | | Cooking Time: 40 Minutes | Servings: 2 |
|---|---|---|---|

| | | |
|---|---|---|
| ✓ 6-ounce cooked salmon, chopped<br>✓ 1 tbsp fresh dill, chopped<br>✓ Salt and black pepper, to taste<br>✓ 2 celery stalks, chopped | ✓ 4 hard-boiled grass-fed eggs, peeled and cubed<br>✓ ½ yellow onion, chopped<br>✓ ¾ cup avocado mayonnaise | ❖ Put all the ingredients in a bowl and mix until well combined.<br>❖ Cover with a plastic wrap and refrigerate for about 3 hours to serve.<br>❖ For meal prepping, put the salad in a container and refrigerate for up to days |

## 117)  BEEF SAUTEED WITH MOROCCAN SPICES AND BUTTERNUT SQUASH WITH CHICKPEAS

| | | Cooking Time: 15 Minutes | Servings: 4 |
|---|---|---|---|

| | | |
|---|---|---|
| ✓ 1 tbsp olive oil, plus 2 tsp<br>✓ 1 pound precut butternut squash cut into ½-inch cubes<br>✓ 3 ounces scallions, white and green parts chopped (1 cup)<br>✓ 1 tbsp water<br>✓ ¼ tsp baking soda<br>✓ ¾ pound flank steak, sliced across the grain into ⅛-inch thick slices<br>✓ ½ tsp garlic powder<br>✓ ¼ tsp ground ginger<br>✓ ¼ tsp turmeric | ✓ ¼ tsp ground cumin<br>✓ ¼ tsp ground coriander<br>✓ ⅛ tsp cayenne pepper<br>✓ ⅛ tsp ground cinnamon<br>✓ ½ tsp kosher salt, divided<br>✓ 1 (14-ounce) can chickpeas, drained and rinsed<br>✓ ½ cup dried apricots, quartered<br>✓ ½ cup cilantro leaves, chopped<br>✓ 2 tsp freshly squeezed lemon juice<br>✓ 8 tsp sliced almonds | ❖ Heat tbsp of oil in a 12-inch skillet. Once the oil is hot, add the squash and scallions, and cook until the squash is tender, about 10 to 12 minutes.<br>❖ Mix the water and baking soda together in a small prep bowl. Place the beef in a medium bowl, pour the baking-soda water over it, and mix to combine. Let it sit for 5 minutes.<br>❖ In a small bowl, combine the garlic powder, ginger, turmeric, cumin, coriander, cayenne, cinnamon, and ¼ tsp of salt, then add the mixture to the beef. Stir to combine.<br>❖ When the squash is tender, turn the heat off and add the remaining ¼ tsp of salt and the chickpeas, dried apricots, cilantro, and lemon juice to taste. Stir to combine. Place the contents of the pan in a bowl to cool.<br>❖ Clean out the skillet and heat the remaining 2 tsp of oil over high heat. When the oil is hot, add the beef and cook until it is no longer pink, about 2 to 3 minutes.<br>❖ Place 1¼ cups of the squash mixture and one quarter of the beef slices in each of 4 containers. Sprinkle 2 tsp of sliced almonds over each container.<br>❖ STORAGE: Store covered containers in the refrigerator for up to 5 days. |

## 118) NORTH AFRICAN–INSPIRED SAUTÉED SHRIMP AND LEEKS WITH PEPPERS

| | Cooking Time: 20 Minutes | Servings: 4 |
|---|---|---|

**Ingredients:**

- ✓ 2 tbsp olive oil, divided
- ✓ 1 large leek, white and light green parts, halved lengthwise, sliced ¼-inch thick
- ✓ 2 tsp chopped garlic
- ✓ 1 large red bell pepper, chopped into ¼-inch pieces
- ✓ 1 cup chopped fresh parsley leaves (1 small bunch)
- ✓ ½ cup chopped fresh cilantro leaves (½ small bunch)
- ✓ ¼ tsp ground cumin
- ✓ ¼ tsp ground coriander
- ✓ 1 tsp smoked paprika
- ✓ 1 pound uncooked peeled, deveined large shrimp (20 to 25 per pound), thawed if frozen, blotted with paper towels
- ✓ 1 tbsp freshly squeezed lemon juice
- ✓ ⅛ tsp kosher salt

**Directions:**

- ❖ Heat 2 tsp of oil in a -inch skillet over medium heat. Once the oil is hot, add the leeks and garlic and sauté for 2 minutes. Add the peppers and cook for 10 minutes, or until the peppers are soft, stirring occasionally.
- ❖ Add the chopped parsley and cilantro and cook for 1 more minute. Remove the mixture from the pan and place in a medium bowl.
- ❖ Mix the cumin, coriander, and paprika in a small prep bowl.
- ❖ Add 2 tsp of oil to the same skillet and increase the heat to medium-high. Add the shrimp in a single layer, sprinkle the spice mixture over the shrimp, and cook for about 2 minutes. Flip the shrimp over and cook for 1 more minute. Add the leek and herb mixture, stir, and cook for 1 more minute.
- ❖ Turn off the heat and add the remaining 2 tsp of oil and the lemon juice. Taste to see whether you need the salt. Add if necessary.
- ❖ Place ¾ cup of couscous or other grain (if using) and 1 cup of the shrimp mixture in each of 4 containers.
- ❖ STORAGE: Store covered containers in the refrigerator for up to 4 days.

## 119) Italian-style Chicken With Sweet Potato And Broccoli

| | Cooking Time: 30 Minutes | Servings: 8 |
|---|---|---|

- ✓ 2 lbs boneless skinless chicken breasts, cut into small pieces
- ✓ 5-6 cups broccoli florets
- ✓ 3 tbsp Italian seasoning mix of your choice
- ✓ a few tbsp of olive oil
- ✓ 3 sweet potatoes, peeled and diced
- ✓ Coarse sea salt, to taste
- ✓ Freshly cracked pepper, to taste
- ✓ Toppings:
- ✓ Avocado
- ✓ Lemon juice
- ✓ Chives
- ✓ Olive oil, for serving

**Directions:**

- ❖ Preheat the oven to 425 degrees F
- ❖ Toss the chicken pieces with the Italian seasoning mix and a drizzle of olive oil, stir to combine then store in the fridge for about 30 minutes
- ❖ Arrange the broccoli florets and sweet potatoes on a sheet pan, drizzle with the olive oil, sprinkle generously with salt
- ❖ Arrange the chicken on a separate sheet pan
- ❖ Bake both in the oven for 12-1minutes
- ❖ Transfer the chicken and broccoli to a plate, toss the sweet potatoes and continue to roast for another 15 minutes, or until ready
- ❖ Allow the chicken, broccoli, and sweet potatoes to cool
- ❖ Distribute among the containers and store for 2-3 days
- ❖ To Serve: Reheat in the microwave for 1 minute or until heated through, top with the topping of choice. Enjoy
- ❖ Recipe Notes: Any kind of vegetables work will with this recipe! So, add favorites like carrots, brussels sprouts and asparagus.

**Nutrition:** Calories:222;Total Fat: 4.9g;Total Carbs: 15.3g;Protein: 28g

## 120) VEGETABLE SOUP

| | Cooking Time: 20 Minutes | Servings: 6 |
|---|---|---|

**Ingredients:**

- ✓ 1 15-ounce can low sodium cannellini beans, drained and rinsed
- ✓ 1 tbsp olive oil
- ✓ 1 small onion, diced
- ✓ 2 carrots, diced
- ✓ 2 stalks celery, diced
- ✓ 1 small zucchini, diced
- ✓ 1 garlic clove, minced
- ✓ 1 tbsp fresh thyme leaves, chopped
- ✓ 2 tsp fresh sage, chopped
- ✓ ½ tsp salt
- ✓ ¼ tsp freshly ground black pepper
- ✓ 32 ounces low sodium chicken broth
- ✓ 1 14-ounce can no-salt diced tomatoes, undrained
- ✓ 2 cups baby spinach leaves, chopped
- ✓ 1/3 cup freshly grated parmesan

**Directions:**

- ❖ Mash half of the beans in a small bowl using the back of a spoon and put it to the side.
- ❖ Add the oil to a large soup pot and place over medium-high heat.
- ❖ Add carrots, onion, celery, garlic, zucchini, thyme, salt, pepper, and sage.
- ❖ Cook well for about 5 minutes until the vegetables are tender.
- ❖ Add broth and tomatoes and bring the mixture to a boil.
- ❖ Add beans (both mashed and whole) and spinach.
- ❖ Cook for 3 minutes until the spinach has wilted.
- ❖ Pour the soup into the jars.
- ❖ Before serving, top with parmesan.
- ❖ Enjoy!

**Nutrition:** Calories: 359, Total Fat: 7.1 g, Saturated Fat: 2.7 g, Cholesterol: 10 mg, Sodium: 854 mg, Total Carbohydrate: 51.1 g, Dietary Fiber: 20 g, Total Sugars: 5.7 g, Protein: 25.8 g, Vitamin D: 0 mcg, Calcium: 277 mg, Iron: 7 mg, Potassium: 1497 mg

## 121) GREEK-STYLE CHICKEN WRAPS

| | Cooking Time: 15 Minutes | Servings: 2 |
|---|---|---|

**Ingredients:**

- ✓ Greek Chicken Wrap Filling:
- ✓ 2 chicken breasts 14 oz, chopped into 1-inch pieces
- ✓ 2 small zucchinis, cut into 1-inch pieces
- ✓ 2 bell peppers, cut into 1-inch pieces
- ✓ 1 red onion, cut into 1-inch pieces
- ✓ 2 tbsp olive oil
- ✓ 2 tsp oregano
- ✓ 2 tsp basil
- ✓ 1/2 tsp garlic powder
- ✓ 1/2 tsp onion powder
- ✓ 1/2 tsp salt
- ✓ 2 lemons, sliced
- ✓ To Serve:
- ✓ 1/4 cup feta cheese crumbled
- ✓ 4 large flour tortillas or wraps

**Directions:**

- ❖ Pre-heat oven to 425 degrees F
- ❖ In a bowl, toss together the chicken, zucchinis, olive oil, oregano, basil, garlic, bell peppers, onion powder, onion powder and salt
- ❖ Arrange lemon slice on the baking sheet(s), spread the chicken and vegetable out on top (use 2 baking sheets if needed)
- ❖ Bake for 15 minutes, until veggies are soft and the chicken is cooked through Allow to cool completely
- ❖ Distribute the chicken, bell pepper, zucchini and onions among the containers and remove the lemon slices Allow the dish to cool completely
- ❖ Distribute among the containers, store for 3 days
- ❖ To Serve: Reheat in the microwave for 1-2 minutes or until heated through. Wrap in a tortila and sprinkle with feta cheese. Enjoy

**Nutrition:** (1 wrap): Calories:356;Total Fat: 14g;Total Carbs: 26g;Protein: 29g

## 122)  GARBANZO BEAN SOUP

| Cooking Time: 20 Minutes | Servings: 4 |
|---|---|

| Ingredients | | Instructions |
|---|---|---|
| ✓ 14 ounces diced tomatoes <br> ✓ 1 tsp olive oil <br> ✓ 1 15-ounce can garbanzo beans | ✓ salt <br> ✓ pepper <br> ✓ 2 sprigs fresh rosemary <br> ✓ 1 cup acini di pepe pasta | ❖ Take a large saucepan and add tomatoes and ounces of the beans. <br> ❖ Bring the mixture to a boil over medium-high heat. <br> ❖ Puree the remaining beans in a blender/food processor. <br> ❖ Stir the pureed mixture into the pan. <br> ❖ Add the sprigs of rosemary to the pan. <br> ❖ Add acini de Pepe pasta and simmer until the pasta is soft, making sure to stir it from time to time. <br> ❖ Remove the rosemary. <br> ❖ Season with pepper and salt. <br> ❖ Enjoy! |

## 123)  ITALIAN SALAD OF SPINACH AND BEANS

| Cooking Time: 30 Minutes | Servings: 4 |
|---|---|

| Ingredients | | Instructions |
|---|---|---|
| ✓ 15 ounces drained and rinsed cannellini beans <br> ✓ 14 ounces drained, rinsed, and quartered artichoke hearts <br> ✓ 6 ounces or 8 cups baby spinach <br> ✓ 14 ½ ounces undrained diced tomatoes, no salt is best <br> ✓ 1 tbsp olive oil and any additional if you prefer | ✓ ¼ tsp salt <br> ✓ 2 minced garlic cloves <br> ✓ 1 chopped onion, small in size <br> ✓ ¼ tsp pepper <br> ✓ ⅛ tsp crushed red pepper flakes <br> ✓ 2 tbsp Worcestershire sauce | ❖ Place a saucepan on your stovetop and turn the temperature to medium-high. <br> ❖ Let the pan warm up for a minute before you pour in the tbsp of oil. Continue to let the oil heat up for another minute or two. <br> ❖ Toss in your chopped onion and stir so all the pieces are bathed in oil. Saute the onions for minutes. <br> ❖ Add the garlic to the saucepan. Stir and saute the ingredients for another minute. <br> ❖ Combine the salt, red pepper flakes, pepper, and Worcestershire sauce. Mix well and then add the tomatoes to the pan. Stir the mixture constantly for about minutes. <br> ❖ Add the artichoke hearts, spinach, and beans. Saute and stir occasionally to get the taste throughout the dish. Once the spinach starts to wilt, take the salad off of the heat. <br> ❖ Serve and enjoy immediately to get the best taste. |

## 124)  SALMON SKILLET LUNCH

| Cooking Time: 15 To 20 Minutes | Servings: 4 |
|---|---|

| Ingredients | | Instructions |
|---|---|---|
| ✓ 1 tsp minced garlic <br> ✓ 1 ½ cup quartered cherry tomatoes <br> ✓ 1 tbsp water <br> ✓ ¼ tsp sea salt <br> ✓ 1 tbsp lemon juice, freshly squeezed is best | ✓ 1 tbsp extra virgin olive oil <br> ✓ 12 ounces drained and chopped roasted red peppers <br> ✓ 1 tsp paprika <br> ✓ ¼ tsp black pepper <br> ✓ 1 pound salmon fillets | ❖ Remove the skin from your salmon fillets and cut them into 8 pieces. <br> ❖ Turn your stove burner on medium heat and set a skillet on top. Pour the olive oil into the skillet and let it heat up for a couple of minutes. <br> ❖ Add the minced garlic and paprika. Saute the ingredients for 1 minute. <br> ❖ Combine the roasted peppers, black pepper, tomatoes, water, and salt. <br> ❖ Set the heat to medium-high and bring the ingredients to a simmer. This should take 3 to 4 minutes. Remember to stir the ingredients occasionally so the tomatoes don't burn. Add the salmon and take some of the sauce from the skillet to spoon on top of the fish so it is all covered in the mixture. <br> ❖ Cover the skillet and set a timer for 10 minutes. When the fish reaches 145 degrees Fahrenheit, it is cooked thoroughly. Turn off the heat and drizzle lemon juice over the fish. <br> ❖ Break up the salmon into chunks and gently mix the pieces of fish with the sauce. Serve and enjoy! |

# Chapter 3. DINNER

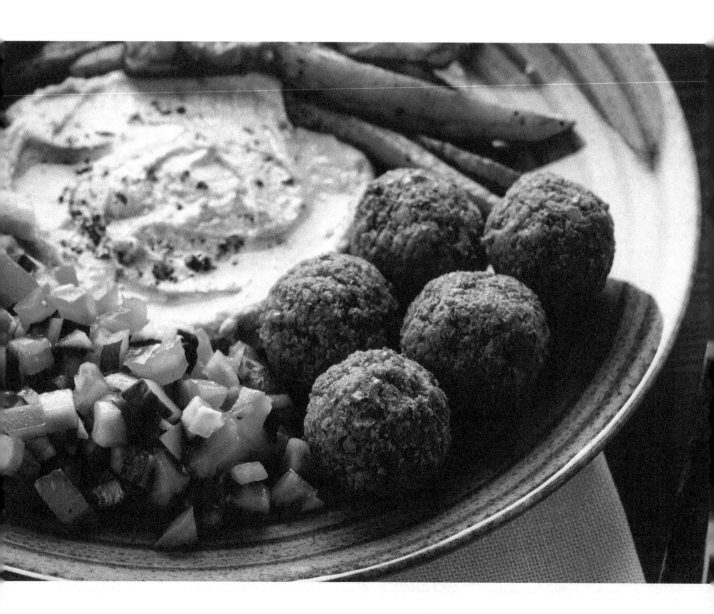

## 125) LEMON FISH GRILL

| | Cooking Time: 15 Minutes | Servings: 4 |
|---|---|---|

**Ingredients:**

✓ ¼ tsp sea salt
✓ 3 to 4 lemons
✓ ¼ tsp ground black pepper
✓ 4 ounces any fish fillets, such as salmon or cod
✓ 1 tbsp olive oil

**Directions:**

❖ Ensure that the fish fillets are dry. If you know or feel they are a bit damp, take a paper towel and pat them dry.

❖ Leave the fish fillets on the counter for 10 minutes so they can stand at room temperature.

❖ Turn on your grill to medium-high heat or set the temperature to 400 degrees Fahrenheit.

❖ Using nonstick cooking spray, coat the grill so the fish won't stick.

❖ Take one lemon and cut it in half. Set one of the halves aside and cut the remaining half into ¼-inch thick slices.

❖ Now, take the other half of the lemon and squeeze at least 1 tbsp of juice out into a small bowl.

❖ Add oil into the small bowl and whisk the ingredients together.

❖ Brush the fish with the lemon and oil mixture. Make sure you get both sides of the fish.

❖ Arrange the lemon slices on the grill in the shape of the fish, it might take about 3 to 4 slices for one fish.

❖ Place the fish on top of the lemon slices and grill the ingredients together. If you don't have a lid for your grill, cover it with a different lid that will fit or use aluminum foil.

❖ When the fish is about half-way done, turn it over so the other side is laying on top of the lemon slices.

❖ You will know the fish is done when it starts to look flaky and separates easily, which you can check by gently pressing a fork onto the fish.

**Nutrition:** calories: 147, fats: 5 grams, carbohydrates: 4 grams, protein: 22 grams.

## 126) BAKED BEANS ITALIAN STYLE

| | Cooking Time: 15 To 20 Minutes. | Servings: 6 |
|---|---|---|

**Ingredients:**

✓ ½ cup chopped onion
✓ ¼ cup red wine vinegar
✓ ¼ tbsp ground cinnamon
✓ 15 ounces or 2 cans of great northern beans, do not drain
✓ 2 tsp extra virgin olive oil
✓ 12 ounces tomato paste, low sodium
✓ ½ cup water

**Directions:**

❖ Turn a burner to medium heat and add oil to a saucepan.

❖ Add the onion and cook for 4 to 5 minutes. Stir well.

❖ Combine the vinegar, tomato paste, cinnamon, and water. Mix until all the ingredients are well combined.

❖ Switch the heat to a low setting.

❖ Using a colander, drain one can of beans and pour into the pan.

❖ Open the second can of beans and pour all of it, including the liquid, into the saucepan and stir.

❖ Continue to cook the beans for 10 minutes while stirring frequently.

❖ Serve and enjoy!

**Nutrition:** calories: 236, fats: 3 grams, carbohydrates: 42 grams, protein: 10 grams

| 127) POMODORO TILAPIA | | |
|---|---|---|
| **Cooking Time:** 15 Minutes | | **Servings: 4** |
| ✓ 3 tbsp sun-dried tomatoes packed in oil, drained (juice/oil reserved) and chopped<br>✓ 1 tbsp capers, drained<br>✓ 2 pieces tilapia | ✓ 1 tbsp oil from sun-dried tomatoes<br>✓ 1 tbsp lemon juice<br>✓ 2 tbsp Kalamata olives, pitted and chopped | ❖ Preheat oven to 375 degrees F.<br>❖ Add sun-dried tomatoes, capers, and olives to a bowl; stir well and set aside.<br>❖ Place the tilapia fillets side by side on a baking sheet.<br>❖ Drizzle with oil and lemon juice.<br>❖ Bake for about 10-1minutes.<br>❖ Check the fish after 10 minutes to see if they are flakey.<br>❖ Once done, top the fish with tomato mixture. |

| 128) LENTIL SOUP WITH CHICKEN | | |
|---|---|---|
| **Cooking Time:** 45 Minutes | | **Servings: 4** |
| ✓ 1 pound dried lentils<br>✓ 12 ounces boneless chicken thigh meat<br>✓ 7 cups water<br>✓ 1 small onion, diced<br>✓ 2 scallions, chopped<br>✓ ¼ cup chopped cilantro | ✓ 3 cloves garlic<br>✓ 1 medium tomato, diced<br>✓ 1 tsp garlic powder<br>✓ 1 tsp cumin<br>✓ ¼ tsp oregano<br>✓ ½ tsp paprika<br>✓ ½ tsp kosher salt | ❖ Add all of the listed Ingredients: to your Instant Pot.<br>❖ Set your pot to SOUP mode and cook for 30 minutes.<br>❖ Allow the pressure to release naturally.<br>❖ Take the chicken out and shred.<br>❖ Place the chicken back in the pot and stir.<br>❖ Pour to the jars.<br>❖ Enjoy! |

| 129) ASPARAGUS WRAPPED WITH BACON | | |
|---|---|---|
| **Cooking Time:** 30 Minutes | | **Servings: 2** |
| **Ingredients:**<br>✓ 1/3 cup heavy whipping cream<br>✓ 2 bacon slices, precooked | ✓ 4 small spears asparagus<br>✓ Salt, to taste<br>✓ 1 tbsp butter | ❖ Preheat the oven to 360 degrees F and grease a baking sheet with butter.<br>❖ Meanwhile, mix cream, asparagus and salt in a bowl.<br>❖ Wrap the asparagus in bacon slices and arrange them in the baking dish.<br>❖ Transfer the baking dish in the oven and bake for about 20 minutes.<br>❖ Remove from the oven and serve hot.<br>❖ Place the bacon wrapped asparagus in a dish and set aside to cool for meal prepping. Divide it in 2 containers and cover the lid. Refrigerate for about 2 days and reheat in the microwave before serving. |

| 130) COOL ITALIAN-STYLE FISH | | |
|---|---|---|
| **Cooking Time:** 30 Minutes | | **Servings: 8** |
| ✓ 6 ounces halibut fillets<br>✓ 1 tbsp Greek seasoning<br>✓ 1 large tomato, chopped<br>✓ 1 onion, chopped<br>✓ 5 ounces kalamata olives, pitted | ✓ ¼ cup capers<br>✓ ¼ cup olive oil<br>✓ 1 tbsp lemon juice<br>✓ Salt and pepper as needed | ❖ Pre-heat your oven to 350-degree Fahrenheit<br>❖ Transfer the halibut fillets on a large aluminum foil Season with Greek seasoning<br>❖ Take a bowl and add tomato, onion, olives, olive oil, capers, pepper, lemon juice and salt<br>❖ Mix well and spoon the tomato mix over the halibut Seal the edges and fold to make a packet Place the packet on a baking sheet and bake in your oven for 30-40 minutes Serve once the fish flakes off and enjoy!<br>❖ Meal Prep/Storage Options: Store in airtight containers in your fridge for 1-2 days. |

## 131) FANCY LUNCHEON SALAD

| | | |
|---|---|---|
| | **Cooking Time:** 40 Minutes | **Servings: 2** |

| | | |
|---|---|---|
| ✓ 6-ounce cooked salmon, chopped<br>✓ 1 tbsp fresh dill, chopped<br>✓ Salt and black pepper, to taste | ✓ 4 hard-boiled grass-fed eggs, peeled and cubed<br>✓ 2 celery stalks, chopped<br>✓ ½ yellow onion, chopped<br>✓ ¾ cup avocado mayonnaise | ❖ Put all the ingredients in a bowl and mix until well combined.<br>❖ Cover with a plastic wrap and refrigerate for about 3 hours to serve.<br>❖ For meal prepping, put the salad in a container and refrigerate for up to days |

## 132) BEEF SAUTEED WITH MOROCCAN SPICES AND BUTTERNUT SQUASH WITH CHICKPEAS

| | | |
|---|---|---|
| | **Cooking Time:** 15 Minutes | **Servings: 4** |

| | | |
|---|---|---|
| ✓ 1 tbsp olive oil, plus 2 tsp<br>✓ 1 pound precut butternut squash cut into ½-inch cubes<br>✓ 3 ounces scallions, white and green parts chopped (1 cup)<br>✓ 1 tbsp water<br>✓ ¼ tsp baking soda<br>✓ ¾ pound flank steak, sliced across the grain into ⅛-inch thick slices<br>✓ ½ tsp garlic powder<br>✓ ¼ tsp ground ginger<br>✓ ¼ tsp turmeric | ✓ ¼ tsp ground cumin<br>✓ ¼ tsp ground coriander<br>✓ ⅛ tsp cayenne pepper<br>✓ ⅛ tsp ground cinnamon<br>✓ ½ tsp kosher salt, divided<br>✓ 1 (14-ounce) can chickpeas, drained and rinsed<br>✓ ½ cup dried apricots, quartered<br>✓ ½ cup cilantro leaves, chopped<br>✓ 2 tsp freshly squeezed lemon juice<br>✓ 8 tsp sliced almonds | ❖ Heat tbsp of oil in a 12-inch skillet. Once the oil is hot, add the squash and scallions, and cook until the squash is tender, about 10 to 12 minutes.<br>❖ Mix the water and baking soda together in a small prep bowl. Place the beef in a medium bowl, pour the baking-soda water over it, and mix to combine. Let it sit for 5 minutes.<br>❖ In a small bowl, combine the garlic powder, ginger, turmeric, cumin, coriander, cayenne, cinnamon, and ¼ tsp of salt, then add the mixture to the beef. Stir to combine.<br>❖ When the squash is tender, turn the heat off and add the remaining ¼ tsp of salt and the chickpeas, dried apricots, cilantro, and lemon juice to taste. Stir to combine. Place the contents of the pan in a bowl to cool.<br>❖ Clean out the skillet and heat the remaining 2 tsp of oil over high heat. When the oil is hot, add the beef and cook until it is no longer pink, about 2 to 3 minutes.<br>❖ Place 1¼ cups of the squash mixture and one quarter of the beef slices in each of 4 containers. Sprinkle 2 tsp of sliced almonds over each container.<br>❖ STORAGE: Store covered containers in the refrigerator for up to 5 days. |

## 133) NORTH AFRICAN–INSPIRED SAUTÉED SHRIMP AND LEEKS WITH PEPPERS

| | | |
|---|---|---|
| | **Cooking Time:** 20 Minutes | **Servings: 4** |

| | | |
|---|---|---|
| ✓ 2 tbsp olive oil, divided<br>✓ 1 large leek, white and light green parts, halved lengthwise, sliced ¼-inch thick<br>✓ 2 tsp chopped garlic<br>✓ 1 large red bell pepper, chopped into ¼-inch pieces<br>✓ 1 cup chopped fresh parsley leaves (1 small bunch)<br>✓ ½ cup chopped fresh cilantro leaves (½ small bunch)<br>✓ ¼ tsp ground cumin | ✓ ¼ tsp ground coriander<br>✓ 1 tsp smoked paprika<br>✓ 1 pound uncooked peeled, deveined large shrimp (20 to 25 per pound), thawed if frozen, blotted with paper towels<br>✓ 1 tbsp freshly squeezed lemon juice<br>✓ ⅛ tsp kosher salt | ❖ Heat 2 tsp of oil in a -inch skillet over medium heat. Once the oil is hot, add the leeks and garlic and sauté for 2 minutes. Add the peppers and cook for 10 minutes, or until the peppers are soft, stirring occasionally.<br>❖ Add the chopped parsley and cilantro and cook for 1 more minute. Remove the mixture from the pan and place in a medium bowl.<br>❖ Mix the cumin, coriander, and paprika in a small prep bowl.<br>❖ Add 2 tsp of oil to the same skillet and increase the heat to medium-high. Add the shrimp in a single layer, sprinkle the spice mixture over the shrimp, and cook for about 2 minutes. Flip the shrimp over and cook for 1 more minute. Add the leek and herb mixture, stir, and cook for 1 more minute.<br>❖ Turn off the heat and add the remaining 2 tsp of oil and the lemon juice. Taste to see whether you need the salt. Add if necessary.<br>❖ Place ¾ cup of couscous or other grain (if using) and 1 cup of the shrimp mixture in each of 4 containers.<br>❖ STORAGE: Store covered containers in the refrigerator for up to 4 days. |

**Nutrition:** Total calories: 1; Total fat: 9g; Saturated fat: 1g; Sodium: 403mg; Carbohydrates: 9g; Fiber: 2g; Protein: 19g

## 134)  ITALIAN-STYLE CHICKEN WITH SWEET POTATO AND BROCCOLI

| | Cooking Time: 30 Minutes | Servings: 8 |
|---|---|---|

**Ingredients:**

- ✓ 2 lbs boneless skinless chicken breasts, cut into small pieces
- ✓ 5-6 cups broccoli florets
- ✓ 3 tbsp Italian seasoning mix of your choice
- ✓ a few tbsp of olive oil
- ✓ 3 sweet potatoes, peeled and diced
- ✓ Coarse sea salt, to taste
- ✓ Freshly cracked pepper, to taste
- ✓ Toppings:
- ✓ Avocado
- ✓ Lemon juice
- ✓ Chives
- ✓ Olive oil, for serving

**Directions:**

- ❖ Preheat the oven to 425 degrees F
- ❖ Toss the chicken pieces with the Italian seasoning mix and a drizzle of olive oil, stir to combine then store in the fridge for about 30 minutes
- ❖ Arrange the broccoli florets and sweet potatoes on a sheet pan, drizzle with the olive oil, sprinkle generously with salt
- ❖ Arrange the chicken on a separate sheet pan
- ❖ Bake both in the oven for 12-1minutes
- ❖ Transfer the chicken and broccoli to a plate, toss the sweet potatoes and continue to roast for another 15 minutes, or until ready
- ❖ Allow the chicken, broccoli, and sweet potatoes to cool
- ❖ Distribute among the containers and store for 2-3 days
- ❖ To Serve: Reheat in the microwave for 1 minute or until heated through, top with the topping of choice. Enjoy
- ❖ Recipe Notes: Any kind of vegetables work will with this recipe! So, add favorites like carrots, brussels sprouts and asparagus.

**Nutrition:** Calories:222;Total Fat: 4.9g;Total Carbs: 15.3g;Protein: 28g

## 135)  VEGETABLE SOUP

| | Cooking Time: 20 Minutes | Servings: 6 |
|---|---|---|

**Ingredients:**

- ✓ 1 15-ounce can low sodium cannellini beans, drained and rinsed
- ✓ 1 tbsp olive oil
- ✓ 1 small onion, diced
- ✓ 2 carrots, diced
- ✓ 2 stalks celery, diced
- ✓ 1 small zucchini, diced
- ✓ 1 garlic clove, minced
- ✓ 1 tbsp fresh thyme leaves, chopped
- ✓ 2 tsp fresh sage, chopped
- ✓ ½ tsp salt
- ✓ ¼ tsp freshly ground black pepper
- ✓ 32 ounces low sodium chicken broth
- ✓ 1 14-ounce can no-salt diced tomatoes, undrained
- ✓ 2 cups baby spinach leaves, chopped
- ✓ 1/3 cup freshly grated parmesan

**Directions:**

- ❖ Mash half of the beans in a small bowl using the back of a spoon and put it to the side.
- ❖ Add the oil to a large soup pot and place over medium-high heat.
- ❖ Add carrots, onion, celery, garlic, zucchini, thyme, salt, pepper, and sage.
- ❖ Cook well for about 5 minutes until the vegetables are tender.
- ❖ Add broth and tomatoes and bring the mixture to a boil.
- ❖ Add beans (both mashed and whole) and spinach.
- ❖ Cook for 3 minutes until the spinach has wilted.
- ❖ Pour the soup into the jars.
- ❖ Before serving, top with parmesan.
- ❖ Enjoy!

## 136) GREEK-STYLE CHICKEN WRAPS

| | Cooking Time: 15 Minutes | Servings: 2 |
|---|---|---|

| | | |
|---|---|---|
| ✓ Greek Chicken Wrap Filling:<br>✓ 2 chicken breasts 14 oz, chopped into 1-inch pieces<br>✓ 2 small zucchinis, cut into 1-inch pieces<br>✓ 2 bell peppers, cut into 1-inch pieces<br>✓ 1 red onion, cut into 1-inch pieces<br>✓ 2 tbsp olive oil | ✓ 2 tsp oregano<br>✓ 2 tsp basil<br>✓ 1/2 tsp garlic powder<br>✓ 1/2 tsp onion powder<br>✓ 1/2 tsp salt<br>✓ 2 lemons, sliced<br>✓ To Serve:<br>✓ 1/4 cup feta cheese crumbled<br>✓ 4 large flour tortillas or wraps | ❖ Pre-heat oven to 425 degrees F<br>❖ In a bowl, toss together the chicken, zucchinis, olive oil, oregano, basil, garlic, bell peppers, onion powder, onion powder and salt<br>❖ Arrange lemon slice on the baking sheet(s), spread the chicken and vegetable out on top (use 2 baking sheets if needed)<br>❖ Bake for 15 minutes, until veggies are soft and the chicken is cooked through Allow to cool completely<br>❖ Distribute the chicken, bell pepper, zucchini and onions among the containers and remove the lemon slices Allow the dish to cool completely<br>❖ Distribute among the containers, store for 3 days<br>❖ To Serve: Reheat in the microwave for 1-2 minutes or until heated through. Wrap in a tortila and sprinkle with feta cheese. Enjoy |

## 137) CLASSIC ITALIAN HERB BREAD

| | Cooking Time: 40 Minutes | Servings: 25 |
|---|---|---|

| | | |
|---|---|---|
| ✓ 1 2/3 tsp active dry yeast<br>✓ 3½ cups all-purpose flour<br>✓ 2 1/4 cup rye flour<br>✓ 1 tbsp salt<br>✓ 2 tbsp olive oil<br>✓ 1 tbsp flat-leaf parsley, finely chopped | ✓ 10 sprigs fresh thyme leaves, stems removed<br>✓ 1 garlic clove, peeled and finely chopped<br>✓ ¼ cup black olives, pitted and chopped<br>✓ 3 green chilies, deseeded and chopped<br>✓ ¾ cup sun-dried tomatoes, drained and chopped | ❖ Take a bowl of lukewarm water (temperature of 0 degrees F) and dissolve 1 and 2/3 cups of yeast.<br>❖ Add flour, yeast water, and salt to another bowl.<br>❖ Mix well to prepare the dough using a mixer or your hands.<br>❖ Put the dough in a large, clean bowl and allow it to rest covered for 2 hours.<br>❖ Transfer dough to a lightly floured surface and knead, adding the parsley, garlic, olives, thyme, tomatoes, and chilies.<br>❖ Place the kneaded dough in an 8½-inch bread-proofing basket.<br>❖ Cover and allow to rest for about 60 minutes.<br>❖ Preheat oven to 400 degrees F.<br>❖ Line a baking sheet with parchment paper.<br>❖ Bake for about 30-40 minutes.<br>❖ Once done, enjoy it! |

## 138) GREEK KIDNEY BEAN, VEGGIE, AND GRAPE SALAD WITH FETA

| | Cooking Time: 25 Minutes | Servings: 4 |
|---|---|---|

| | | |
|---|---|---|
| ✓ 1½ cups red grapes, halved<br>✓ 1 (15-ounce) can red kidney beans, drained and rinsed<br>✓ 10 ounces cherry tomatoes, halved (quartered if tomatoes are large) | ✓ 4 (6-inch) Persian cucumbers, quartered vertically and chopped<br>✓ ½ cup green pumpkin seeds (pepitas)<br>✓ ½ cup feta cheese<br>✓ 2½ ounces baby spinach leaves (about 4 cups)<br>✓ ½ cup Dijon Red Wine Vinaigrette | ❖ Place the grapes, kidney beans, cherry tomatoes, cucumbers, pumpkin seeds, and feta in a large mixing bowl and mix to combine.<br>❖ Place cups of the salad mixture in each of 4 containers. Then place 1 cup of spinach leaves on top of each salad. Pour 2 tbsp of vinaigrette into each of 4 sauce containers. Refrigerate all the containers.<br>❖ STORAGE: Store covered containers in the refrigerator for up to 5 days. |

**Nutrition:** Info:Per Serving: Total calories: 5; Total fat: 25g; Saturated fat: 6g; Sodium: 435mg; Carbohydrates: 37g; Fiber: 10g; Protein: 16g

## 139) ITALIAN SUMAC CHICKPEA BOWL

| | Cooking Time: 25 Minutes | Servings: 4 |
|---|---|---|

**Ingredients:**

- ⅔ cup uncooked bulgur
- 1⅓ cups water
- ⅛ tsp kosher salt
- 1 tsp olive oil
- 2 tbsp olive oil
- 2 (15.5-ounce) cans low-sodium chickpeas, drained and rinsed
- 3 tbsp sumac
- ¼ tsp kosher salt
- 4 Persian cucumbers, quartered lengthwise and chopped (about 2 cups)
- ✓ 10 ounces cherry tomatoes, quartered (halved if you have small tomatoes)
- ✓ ¼ cup chopped fresh mint
- ✓ 1 cup chopped fresh parsley
- ✓ 4 tsp olive oil
- ✓ 2 tbsp plus 2 tsp freshly squeezed lemon juice
- ✓ ¼ tsp kosher salt
- ✓ 2 tbsp unsalted tahini
- ✓ ¼ tsp garlic powder
- ✓ 5 tbsp water

**Directions:**

- ❖ TO MAKE THE BULGUR
- ❖ Place the bulgur, water, and salt in a saucepan, and bring to a boil. Once it boils, cover the pot with a lid and turn off the heat. Let the covered pot stand for minutes. Stir the oil into the cooked bulgur. Cool.
- ❖ Place ½ cup of bulgur in each of 4 microwaveable containers.
- ❖ TO MAKE THE CHICKPEAS
- ❖ Heat the oil in a 12-inch skillet over medium-high heat. Once the oil is shimmering, add the chickpeas, sumac, and salt, and stir to coat. Cook for 2 minutes without stirring. Give the chickpeas a stir and cook for another 2 minutes without stirring. Stir and cook for 2 more minutes.
- ❖ Place ¾ cup of cooled chickpeas in each of the 4 bulgur containers.
- ❖ TO MAKE THE SALAD
- ❖ Combine all the ingredients for the salad in a medium mixing bowl. Taste for salt and lemon, and add more if you need it.
- ❖ Place 1¼ cup of salad in each of 4 containers. These containers will not be reheated.
- ❖ TO MAKE THE TAHINI SAUCE
- ❖ Combine the tahini and garlic powder in a small bowl. Whisk in 1 tbsp of water at a time until all 5 tbsp have been incorporated and a thin sauce has formed. It will thicken as it sits.
- ❖ Place 1 tbsp of tahini sauce in each of 4 small sauce containers.
- ❖ STORAGE: Store covered containers in the refrigerator for up to 5 days. When serving, reheat the bulgur and chickpeas, add them to the salad, and drizzle the tahini sauce over the top.

**Nutrition:** Total calories: 485; Total fat: 19g; Saturated fat: 2g; Sodium: 361mg; Carbohydrates: 67g; Fiber: 19g; Protein: 16g

## 140) ORIGINAL SMOKED SALMON AND LEMON-DILL RICOTTA BENTO BOX

| | Cooking Time: 10 Minutes | Servings: 4 |
|---|---|---|

**Ingredients:**

- FOR THE LEMON-DILL RICOTTA
- 1 (16-ounce) container whole-milk ricotta cheese
- 1 tsp finely grated lemon zest
- 3 tbsp chopped fresh dill
- ✓ FOR THE BENTO BOX
- ✓ 8 ounces smoked salmon
- ✓ 4 (6-inch) Persian cucumbers or 2 small European cucumbers, sliced
- ✓ 2 cups sugar snap peas
- ✓ 4 whole-wheat pitas, each cut into 4 pieces

**Directions:**

- ❖ Mix all the ingredients for the lemon-dill ricotta in a medium bowl.
- ❖ Divide the salmon, cucumbers, and snap peas among 4 containers.
- ❖ Place 1 pita in each of 4 resealable bags.
- ❖ Place ½ cup of ricotta spread in each of separate small containers, since it may release some liquid after a couple of days.
- ❖ STORAGE: Store covered containers in the refrigerator for up to 4 days. Store the pita at room temperature or in the refrigerator.

**Nutrition:** Total calories: 4; Total fat: 20g; Saturated fat: 11g; Sodium: 1,388mg; Carbohydrates: 40g; Fiber: 8g; Protein: 32g

## 141)  ITALIAN-STYLE BAKED TILAPIA WITH ROASTED BABY RED POTATOES

| | Cooking Time:  35 Minutes | Servings: 2 |
|---|---|---|

**Ingredients:**

- ✓ 3 tsp olive oil, divided
- ✓ 1 small yellow onion, very thinly sliced (about 2½ cups)
- ✓ 1 large red bell pepper, thinly sliced (about 2 cups)
- ✓ 10 ounces baby red potatoes, quartered (about 1-inch pieces)
- ✓ ⅜ tsp kosher salt, divided
- ✓ 1 tsp chopped garlic
- ✓ 1 tbsp capers, drained, rinsed, and roughly chopped
- ✓ ¼ cup golden raisins
- ✓ 1 (½-ounce) pack fresh basil, roughly chopped
- ✓ 2½ ounces baby spinach, large leaves torn in half (about 4 cups)
- ✓ 2 tsp freshly squeezed lemon juice
- ✓ 8 ounces tilapia or other thin white fish (see tip)

**Directions:**

- ❖ Preheat the oven to 450°F. Line a sheet pan with a silicone baking mat or parchment paper.
- ❖ Heat tsp of oil in a 12-inch skillet over medium heat. When the oil is shimmering, add the onions and peppers. Cook for 12 minutes, stirring occasionally. The onions should be very soft.
- ❖ While the onions and peppers are cooking, place the potatoes on the sheet pan and toss with ⅛ tsp of salt and the remaining 1 tsp of oil. Spread the potatoes out evenly across half of the pan. Roast in the oven for 10 minutes.
- ❖ Once the onions are soft, add the garlic, capers, raisins, basil, ⅛ tsp of salt, and the spinach. Stir to combine and cook for 3 more minutes to wilt the spinach.
- ❖ Carefully remove the sheet pan from the oven after 10 minutes. Add half of the onion mixture to the empty side of the pan to form a nest for the fish. Place the fish on top and season with the remaining ⅛ tsp of salt and the lemon juice. Spread the rest of the onion mixture evenly across the top of the fish.
- ❖ Place the pan back in the oven and cook for 10 minutes. The fish should be flaky.
- ❖ When the fish and potatoes have cooled, place 1 piece of fish plus half of the potatoes and half of the onion mixture in each of 2 containers. Refrigerate.
- ❖ STORAGE: Store covered containers in the refrigerator for up to 4 days.

## 142)  ITALIAN-STYLE FOCACCIA

| | Cooking Time:  30 Minutes | Servings: 4 |
|---|---|---|

- ✓ 3 3/5 cups flour
- ✓ 1 1/7 cups warm water
- ✓ 2 tbsp olive oil
- ✓ 2 tsp dry yeast
- ✓ 1½ tsp salt
- ✓ 1 cup black olives, pitted and coarsely chopped
- ✓ sea salt
- ✓ olive oil

- ❖ Place flour and yeast in a large bowl.
- ❖ Make a well and pour in water, salt, and oil.
- ❖ Gradually keep mixing until everything is incorporated well.
- ❖ Knead for about 20 minutes.
- ❖ Add black olives and mix well.
- ❖ Form a ball and allow it to rise for about 45 minutes (in a bowl covered with a towel).
- ❖ Once the dough is ready, push air out of it by crushing it using your palm.
- ❖ Roll out the dough onto a floured surface to a thickness of about ½ an inch.
- ❖ Place it on a baking sheet covered with parchment paper, and allow the dough to rise for another 45 minutes.
- ❖ Preheat oven to 425 degrees Fahrenheit.
- ❖ Press fingers into the dough at regular intervals to pierce the dough.
- ❖ When ready to bake, pour a bit of olive oil into the holes and sprinkle with salt.
- ❖ Bake for 20-30 minutes.
- ❖ Enjoy!

**Nutrition:** Calories: 523, Total Fat: 11.7 g, Saturated Fat: 1.7 g, Cholesterol: 0 mg, Sodium: 3495 mg, Total Carbohydrate: 89.4 g, Dietary Fiber: 4.6 g, Total

Sugars: 0.3 g, Protein: 13.8 g, Vitamin D: 0 mcg, Calcium: 50 mg, Iron: 7 mg, Potassium: 124 mg

## 143) LOVELY CHEESY OLIVE BREAD

| | Cooking Time: 15 Minutes | Servings: 8 |
|---|---|---|

| Ingredients | Ingredients | Directions |
|---|---|---|
| ✓ ½ cup softened butter<br>✓ ¼ cup mayo<br>✓ 1 tsp garlic powder<br>✓ 1 tsp onion powder | ✓ 2 cups shredded mozzarella cheese<br>✓ ½ cup chopped black olives<br>✓ 1 loaf of French Bread, halved longways | ❖ Preheat oven to a temperature of 350 degrees Fahrenheit.<br>❖ Stir butter and mayo together in a bowl until it is smooth and creamy.<br>❖ Add onion powder, garlic powder, olives, and cheese and stir.<br>❖ Spread the mixture over French bread.<br>❖ Place bread on a baking sheet and bake for 10-12 minutes.<br>❖ Increase the heat to broil and cook until the cheese has melted and the bread is golden brown.<br>❖ Cool and chill.<br>❖ Pre-heat before eating. |

## 144) BEEFSTEAK MARINATED IN ORIGINAL RED WINE WITH BRUSSELS SPROUTS SALAD

| | Cooking Time: 10 Minutes | Servings: 2 |
|---|---|---|

| FOR THE STEAK | FOR THE BRUSSELS SPROUT SLAW | Directions |
|---|---|---|
| ✓ 8 ounces flank steak, trimmed of visible fat<br>✓ ½ cup red wine<br>✓ 2 tbsp low-sodium soy sauce<br>✓ 1 tbsp olive oil<br>✓ ½ tsp garlic powder | ✓ 8 ounces Brussels sprouts, stemmed, halved, and very thinly sliced<br>✓ 3 tbsp unsalted sunflower seeds<br>✓ 3 tbsp freshly squeezed lemon juice<br>✓ 1 tbsp plus 1 tsp olive oil<br>✓ 2 tbsp dried cranberries<br>✓ ⅛ tsp kosher salt<br>✓ ⅔ cup Artichoke-Olive Compote | ❖ TO MAKE THE STEAK<br>❖ Place all the ingredients for the steak in a gallon-size resealable bag. Allow the steak to marinate overnight or up to hours.<br>❖ Place the oven rack about 6 inches from the heating element. Preheat the oven to the broil setting (use the high setting if you have multiple settings).<br>❖ Cover a sheet pan with foil. Lift the steak out of the marinade and place on top of the foil-lined sheet pan. Place the pan in the oven and cook for to 6 minutes on one side. Flip the steak over to the other side and broil for 4 to 6 minutes more.<br>❖ Remove from the oven and allow to rest for to 10 minutes. Medium-rare will be about 135°F when an instant-read meat thermometer is inserted.<br>❖ On a cutting board, slice the steak thinly against the grain and divide the steak between 2 containers.<br>❖ TO MAKE THE BRUSSELS SPROUT SLAW<br>❖ Combine the Brussels sprouts, sunflower seeds, lemon juice, olive oil, cranberries, and salt in a medium bowl.<br>❖ Place 1 cup of Brussels sprout slaw and ⅓ cup of artichoke-olive compote in each of 2 containers. The slaw and compote are meant to be eaten at room temperature, while the steak can be eaten warm. However, if you want to eat the steak at room temperature as well, all the items can be put in the same container.<br>❖ STORAGE: Store covered containers in the refrigerator for up to 5 days. |

## 145) CENTRE ITALY CITRUS SHRIMP AND AVOCADO SALAD

| Preparation Time: 5 minutes | Cooking Time: 10 minutes | Servings: 3 |
|---|---|---|

| Ingredients: | | Directions: |
|---|---|---|
| ✓ 1 tbsp olive oil<br>✓ 1/2 cup lemon juice<br>✓ 1 cup of orange juice<br>✓ 1/2 tsp stone house seasoning<br>✓ 3 lb shrimp | ✓ 2 tbsp chopped parsley<br>✓ 8 cups salad greens<br>✓ 1/2 cup citrus vinaigrette<br>✓ 1/2 sliced red onion<br>✓ One sliced avocado | ❖ In a bowl, mix orange juice, stone house seasoning, oil, and lemon juice.<br>❖ Transfer the bowl mixture to the heated skillet. Cook for five minutes over medium flame.<br>❖ Stir in shrimps and cook for five more minutes.<br>❖ Sprinkle parsley and set aside. Citrus shrimps are ready.<br>❖ Prepare the Citrus Vinaigrette Dressing as per the instruction given on the package.<br>❖ In a bowl, whisk citrus vinaigrette until it emulsified. Mix salad greens, avocado, shrimps, and onion in a citrus vinaigrette. Serve and enjoy it. |

**Nutrition:** Calories: 430 kcal Fat: 21 g Protein: 48 g Carbs: 12 g Fiber: 3 g

## 146) SIMPLE COUSCOUS WITH SUNDRIED TOMATO AND FETA

| Preparation Time: 12 minutes | Cooking Time: | Servings: 6 |
|---|---|---|

**Ingredients:**

- ✓ 1.25 cups dried couscous
- ✓ 1 tsp powdered vegetable stock
- ✓ 1.25 cups boiled water
- ✓ One chopped garlic clove
- ✓ 14 oz chickpeas
- ✓ 1 tsp coriander powder
- ✓ ½ cup chopped coriander
- ✓ One chopped onion
- ✓ ½ cup chopped parsley
- ✓ 7 oz sun-dried tomato
- ✓ One lemon zest
- ✓ 4 oz arugula lettuce
- ✓ Black pepper
- ✓ 5 tbsp lemon juice
- ✓ 2 oz feta cheese
- ✓ ½ tsp black pepper
- ✓ Salt to taste

**Directions:**

- ❖ In a bowl, combine garlic, chickpeas, stock powder, couscous, and coriander.
- ❖ Add hot water to the bowl and mix well. Cover the bowl and keep it aside for about five minutes.
- ❖ Add sun-dried tomatoes, lemon juice, coriander, rocket, pepper, parsley, salt, onions, and lemon zest and toss well.
- ❖ Sprinkle feta cheese and serve.

**Nutrition:** Calories: 260 kcal Fat: 9.2 g Protein: 10 g Carbs: 39 g Fiber: 5.8 g

## 147) ORIGINAL CHARD AND GARLIC CHICKPEAS

| Preparation Time: 10 minutes | Cooking Time: 10 minutes | Servings: 4 |
|---|---|---|

- ✓ 1 cup chopped sundried tomatoes
- ✓ 1 tbsp olive oil Two minced garlic cloves One sliced shallot Two bunches of chopped Swiss chard
- ✓ 15 oz chickpeas One lemon
- ✓ 1/4 cup vegetable broth

- ❖ Cook shallot in heated oil over medium flame until they turned translucent.
- ❖ After shallots are translucent, stir in garlic and cook for three minutes.
- ❖ Mix chard and broth and cover, and let it simmer for a few minutes.
- ❖ Add lemon juice, sundried tomatoes, lemon zest, and chickpeas and mix to combine. Cook for three minutes.
- ❖ Serve and enjoy.

## 148) EASY ARUGULA SALAD WITH PESTO SHRIMP, PARMESAN, AND WHITE BEANS

| Preparation Time: 35 minutes | Cooking Time: 15 minutes | Servings: 3 |
|---|---|---|

- ✓ 4 tbsp olive oil
- ✓ 1/2 lb raw shrimp Two minced cloves garlic
- ✓ 1/4 tsp ground black pepper
- ✓ 1/4 tsp salt
- ✓ One pinch of red pepper flakes
- ✓ 1/4 cup pesto Genovese 2 cups cherry tomatoes
- ✓ 8 cups Arugula
- ✓ 1/8 cup grated parmesan cheese
- ✓ 1/2 lemon
- ✓ 1/2 cup white beans

- ❖ In a mixing bowl, add salt, chili flakes, olive oil, shrimp, and black pepper. Mix well and keep it aside for 30 minutes for enhanced flavor.
- ❖ Heat olive oil in a skillet over a high flame. Cook shrimps in oil, two minutes from each side.
- ❖ Lower the flame and stir in tomatoes and garlic. Cook for five more minutes with occasional stirring.
- ❖ Shift cooked shrimps' mixture in a bowl and mix with pesto.
- ❖ In a bowl, mix olive oil, arugula, and lemon juice. Add cheese, tomatoes, salt, beans, and black pepper. Mix well.
- ❖ Serve arugula mixture with cooked shrimps.

**Nutrition:** Calories: 276 kcal Fat: 6.7 g Protein: 30 g Carbs: 23.3 g Fiber: 5.5 g

## 149)  CANTALOUPE AND MOZZARELLA CAPRESE SALAD

| Preparation Time: 10 minutes | Cooking Time: 0 minute | Servings: 8 |
|---|---|---|

**Ingredients:**

- ✓ 1 tbsp white wine vinegar sliced cantaloupes
- ✓ Eight shredded prosciutto
- ✓ 8 oz mozzarella balls
- ✓ ¼ cup chopped basil leaves tbsp extra-virgin olive oil
- ✓ ¼ cup chopped mint leaves
- ✓ Salt to taste
- ✓ 1.5 tbsp honey
- ✓ Black pepper to taste

**Directions:**

- ❖ Take cantaloupe balls out of cantaloupe using melon baller and place in a bowl.
- ❖ Add mozzarella cheese ball, prosciutto, basil, and mint leaves. Mix well.
- ❖ In another bowl, mix honey, vinegar, and olive oil. Pour the dressing over a cantaloupe mixture and mix well.
- ❖ Serve and enjoy it.

**Nutrition:** Calories: 232 kcal Fat: 15 g Protein: 10 g Carbs: 17 g Fiber: 2 g

## 150)  SIMPLE ARUGULA SALAD

| Preparation Time: 5 minutes | Cooking Time: 0 minute | Servings: 2 |
|---|---|---|

**Ingredients:**

- ✓ 4 cups arugula tbsp olive oil
- ✓ 1/2 tsp kosher salt tbsp lemon juice
- ✓ 1/2 tsp black pepper
- ✓ 1/4 cup grated parmesan cheese
- ✓ 1 tsp honey

**Directions:**

- ❖ Combine honey, black pepper, parmesan cheese, olive oil, salt, arugula, and lemon juice. Toss to coat well.
- ❖ Serve and enjoy.

**Nutrition:** Calories: 203 kcal Fat: 18 g Protein: 6 g Carbs: 6 g Fiber: 1 g

## 151)  ITALIAN-STYLE QUINOA SALAD

| Preparation Time: 15 minutes | Cooking Time: 0 minute | Servings: 4 |
|---|---|---|

**Ingredients:**

- ✓ 1.5 cups dry quinoa
- ✓ 1/2 tsp kosher salt
- ✓ 1/2 cup extra virgin olive oil
- ✓ 1 tbsp balsamic vinegar minced garlic cloves
- ✓ 1/2 tsp minced basil
- ✓ 1/2 tsp crushed thyme
- ✓ Black pepper to taste cups arugula
- ✓ 15 oz garbanzo
- ✓ One package salad savors for toppings

**Directions:**

- ❖ In a pot, add water, salt, and quinoa. Cook until quinoa is done. Drain and set aside.
- ❖ Whisk garlic, pepper, thyme, olive oil, salt, basil, and vinegar in a bowl. The dressing is ready. Keep it aside.
- ❖ In a big sized bowl, combine salad savor content, arugula, quinoa, and beans.
- ❖ Pour dressing over the arugula mixture and serve after sprinkling basil over it.

**Nutrition:** Calories: 583 kcal Fat: 33 g Protein: 15 g Carbs: 58 g Fiber: 10 g

## 152) GREEK-STYLE PASTA SALAD WITH CUCUMBER AND ARTICHOKE HEARTS

| Preparation Time: 5 minutes | Cooking Time: 0 minute | Servings: 10 |
| --- | --- | --- |

**Ingredients:**

- ✓ ½ cup olive oil
- ✓ Four minced garlic cloves
- ✓ 1/4 cup white balsamic vinegar tbsp oregano
- ✓ 1 cup crumbled feta cheese
- ✓ 1 tsp ground pepper
- ✓ 15 oz sliced artichoke hearts
- ✓ 1 lb pasta noodles cooked

- ✓ 12 oz roasted and chopped red bell peppers
- ✓ One sliced English cucumber
- ✓ 8 oz sliced Kalamata olives
- ✓ ¼ sliced red onion
- ✓ 1/3 cup chopped basil leaves
- ✓ 1 tsp kosher salt

**Directions:**

- ❖ Combine vinegar, oregano, salt, olive oil, garlic, and black pepper in a bowl and mix well. Set aside.
- ❖ In a big sized bowl, combine olives, onions, cheese, artichoke hearts, cooked pasta, cucumber and bell peppers,
- ❖ Drizzle dressing over the artichoke hearts mixture and toss to coat. Garnish with feta cheese and basil and serve after half an hour.

**Nutrition:** Calories: 415.43 kcal Fat: 23.15 g Protein: 9.54 g Carbs: 42.54 g Fiber: 4.46 g

## 153) SPECIAL QUINOA AND KALE PROTEIN POWER SALAD

| Preparation Time: 5 minutes | Cooking Time: 15 minutes | Servings: 5 |
| --- | --- | --- |

**Ingredients:**

- ✓ One sliced zucchini
- ✓ ½ tbsp extra virgin olive oil
- ✓ ¼ tsp turmeric
- ✓ ¼ tsp cumin
- ✓ ¼ tsp paprika tsp minced garlic,

- ✓ One pinch of red pepper flakes
- ✓ ½ cup cooked quinoa
- ✓ Salt to taste
- ✓ 1 cup drained chickpeas
- ✓ 1 cup chopped curly kale

**Directions:**

- ❖ In a bowl, whisk chili flakes, cumin, paprika, salt, olive oil, garlic, and turmeric. Keep it aside.
- ❖ Toast quinoa for one minute in olive oil.
- ❖ Cook toasted quinoa following the instructions given over the package. Set aside.
- ❖ Sauté garlic, kale, chickpeas, and zucchini in heated olive oil in the same skillet used to toast quinoa.
- ❖ Cook for a few minutes until the mixture starts to sweat. Sprinkle salt and remove skillet from flame.
- ❖ In a bowl, combine veggies mixture and quinoa and leave for 10 minutes.
- ❖ In a skillet, sauté spices in oil for two minutes and add in veggies mixture.
- ❖ Serve and enjoy.

**Nutrition:** Calories: 106 kcal Fat: 3 g Protein: 5 g Carbs: 16 g Fiber: 4 g

## 154)   ITALIAN ANTIPASTO SALAD PLATTER

| Preparation Time: 20 minutes | Cooking Time: 0 minute | Servings: 4 |
|---|---|---|

**Ingredients:**

- ✓ ½ chopped red bell pepper
- ✓ One chopped garlic clove
- ✓ 12 sliced black olive
- ✓ ¼ cup olive oil
- ✓ 2 tbsp balsamic vinegar
- ✓ 1 tbsp chopped basil
- ✓ Black pepper to taste
- ✓ 6 oz artichoke hearts
- ✓ 5 oz Italian blend
- ✓ Salt to taste
- ✓ 1 cup broccoli florets
- ✓ ½ cup sliced onion
- ✓ Eight strawberry tomatoes 3 oz salami dried 4 oz mozzarella cheese

**Directions:**

- ❖ In a mixing bowl, mix salt, vinegar, olive oil, black pepper, garlic, and basil. The dressing is ready.
- ❖ Whisk vinaigrette and salad blend in a bowl.
- ❖ Transfer the salad blend mixture to a platter and organize all the leftover ingredients on the platter and serve.

**Nutrition:** Calories: 351 kcal Fat: 25.9 g Protein: 16.2 g Carbs: 14.8 g Fiber: 3.8 g

## 155)   GREEK STYLE WHOLE WHEAT PASTA SALAD

| Preparation Time: 15 minutes | Cooking Time: 0 minute | Servings: 6 |
|---|---|---|

**Ingredients:**

- ✓ 1 lb rotini pasta
- ✓ One chopped cucumber
- ✓ 1 cup sliced cherry tomatoes
- ✓ One chopped yellow capsicum
- ✓ 1 cup chopped Kalamata olives
- ✓ One diced red onion 2 tbsp chopped dill
- ✓ ½ cup feta cheese
- ✓ Salt to taste
- ✓ Black pepper to taste
- ✓ Dressing
- ✓ 2minced garlic cloves
- ✓ ¼ cup olive oil
- ✓ 3tbsp red wine vinegar
- ✓ ½ lemon juice
- ✓ Salt to taste
- ✓ ½ tsp oregano
- ✓ Black pepper to taste

**Directions:**

- ❖ Bring water to boil in a pot. Stir in salt and cook pasta in it until it is done.
- ❖ Strain pasta and set aside.
- ❖ Mix Olive oil, vinegar, salt, lemon juice, oregano, pepper, and garlic in a bowl. The dressing is ready.
- ❖ Combine cooked pasta, cucumber, olives, feta cheese, onions, bell pepper, tomatoes, and dill in a salad serving bowl.
- ❖ Drizzle dressing over the mixture and toss to coat.
- ❖ Serve and enjoy it.

**Nutrition:** Calories: 437 kcal Fat: 16 g Protein: 14 g Carbs: 64 g Fiber: 2 g

## 156) GREEK-STYLE SALAD

| Preparation Time: 20 minutes | Cooking Time: 0 minute | Servings: 5 |
|---|---|---|

**Ingredients:**

- Dressing
- 6 tbsp olive oil
- ¾ tsp honey
- 1 tbsp red wine vinegar
- 1/5 tbsp lemon juice
- 1.5 tsp minced garlic
- 1 tsp oregano
- 1.5 tbsp minced parsley
- Salt to taste
- Salad
- Four diced tomatoes
- ½ chopped onion
- One chopped English cucumber
- One chopped green bell pepper
- 4 oz feta cheese
- ¾ cup sliced Kalamata olives
- One chopped avocado

**Directions:**

- Whisk all the ingredients mentioned in the dressing list in a large mixing bowl. Set aside.
- In another bowl, add all the ingredients of the salad and toss well.
- Pour the dressing, toss well and serve.

**Nutrition:** Calories: 248 kcal Fat: 24 g Protein: 3 g Carbs: 4 g Fiber: 1 g

## 157) LOVELY CREAMIEST HUMMUS

| Preparation Time: 5 minutes | Cooking Time: 0 minute | Servings: 10 |
|---|---|---|

**Ingredients:**

- 400 g chickpeas
- ½ tsp salt
- 8 tbsp tahini
- 10 tbsp liquid from chickpeas can
- 2 tbsp lemon juice
- 1 tbsp olive oil

**Directions:**

- In a food processor, blend chickpeas, lemon juice, tahini, salt, and aquafaba to get smooth hummus.
- Transfer the blended hummus to the bowl. Pour olive oil in the center of the hummus and serve.

**Nutrition:** Calories: 100 kcal Fat: 7 g Protein: 3 g Carbs: 5 g Fiber: 3 g

## 158) ROASTED ITALIAN VEGETABLES

| Preparation Time: 10 minutes | Cooking Time: 30 minutes | Servings: 6 |
|---|---|---|

**Ingredients:**

- 8 oz mushrooms
- 12 oz Campari tomatoes
- Extra virgin olive as required
- Two sliced zucchinis
- 12 oz sliced baby potatoes
- 11 chopped garlic cloves
- 1 tsp dried thyme
- Salt to taste
- Shredded Parmesan cheese
- Black pepper to taste
- ½ tbsp dried oregano
- Red pepper flakes to taste

**Directions:**

- Add salt, mushrooms, olive oil, pepper, veggies, oregano, garlic, and thyme in a mixing bowl and toss well. Set aside.
- Roast potatoes in a preheated oven at 425 degrees for 10 minutes.
- Mix the mushroom mixture with baked potatoes and bake for another 20 minutes.
- Garnish with cheese and pepper flakes and serve.

**Nutrition:** Calories: 88 kcal Fat: 1 g Protein: 3.8 g Carbs: 14.3 g Fiber: 3.1 g

## 159) PLAIN WHITE BEAN SALAD

| Preparation Time: 15 minutes | Cooking Time: 0 minute | Servings: 4 |
|---|---|---|

**Ingredients:**

- ✓ 2o oz white beans
- ✓ 10 oz halved cherry tomatoes
- ✓ One chopped English cucumber
- ✓ Four chopped onion
- ✓ 18 chopped mint leaves
- ✓ 1 cup chopped parsley
- ✓ 1 tbsp of lemon juice
- ✓ Salt to taste
- ✓ Zested of one lemon
- ✓ Black pepper to taste
- ✓ ½ tsp Sumac
- ✓ Feta cheese
- ✓ 1 tsp Za'atar
- ✓ ½ tsp Aleppo
- ✓ Olive oil

**Directions:**

- ❖ Combine all the ingredients in a large salad bowl and toss well to mix everything evenly.
- ❖ Serve and enjoy it.

**Nutrition:** Calories: 310 kcal Fat: 7 g Protein: 16 g Carbs: 47 g Fiber: 11 g

## 160) EASY ROASTED CAULIFLOWER WITH LEMON AND CUMIN

| Preparation Time: 15 minutes | Cooking Time: 25 minutes | Servings: 4 |
|---|---|---|

- ✓ 11 oz cauliflower
- ✓ 1 tbsp of lemon juice
- ✓ 1/3 cup olive oil
- ✓ Salt to taste
- ✓ Zest of one lemon
- ✓ 1 tbsp ground sumac
- ✓ 1 tbsp ground cumin
- ✓ 1 tsp garlic powder
- ✓ Black pepper to taste

**Directions:**

- ❖ Mix all the ingredients in a large mixing bowl.
- ❖ Transfer the cauliflower to a baking tray and bake in a preheated oven at 425 degrees for 25 minutes.
- ❖ Serve and enjoy it.

## 161) SPECIAL TABBOULEH SALAD

| Preparation Time: 20 minutes | Cooking Time: 0 minute | Servings: 6 |
|---|---|---|

- ✓ ½ cup bulgur wheat
- ✓ One chopped English cucumber
- ✓ Four chopped tomatoes
- ✓ Two chopped parsley
- ✓ Four chopped green onions
- ✓ 13 chopped mint leaves
- ✓ Salt to taste
- ✓ 4 tbsp extra virgin olive oil
- ✓ 4 tbsp lime juice
- ✓ Romaine lettuce leaves to garnishing

**Directions:**

- ❖ Soak bulgur for 10 minutes in water.
- ❖ Drain to remove all the excess water and keep it aside.
- ❖ Now, mix all the ingredients in a large salad bowl and place them for 30 minutes in the refrigerator to get the best results.

**Nutrition:** Calories: 190 kcal Fat: 10 g Protein: 3.2 g Carbs: 25.5 g Fiber: 3.1 g

## 162) TASTY WATERMELON SALAD

| Preparation Time: 15 minutes | Cooking Time: 0 minute | Servings: 6 |
|---|---|---|

**Ingredients:**

- ✓ Honey Vinaigrette
- ✓ 2 tbsp extra virgin olive oil
- ✓ 2 tbsp honey
- ✓ One pinch of salt
- ✓ ½ chopped watermelon
- ✓ Watermelon Salad
- ✓ 2 tbsp lime juice
- ✓ One chopped English cucumber
- ✓ 15 chopped basil leaves
- ✓ 15 chopped mint leaves
- ✓ ½ cup feta cheese

**Directions:**

- ❖ In a bowl, combine watermelon, herbs, and cucumber and set aside.
- ❖ In another bowl, mix oil, salt, honey, and lemon juice and pour the dressing into a watermelon bowl.
- ❖ Toss well and serve.

**Nutrition:** Calories: 192 kcal Fat: 5.6 g Protein: 4.3 g Carbs: 35.9 g Fiber: 11 g

## 163) SPECIAL LOADED CHICKPEA SALAD

| Preparation Time: 20 minutes | Cooking Time: 10 minutes | Servings: 6 |
|---|---|---|

**Ingredients:**

- ✓ Olive oil
- ✓ One sliced eggplant
- ✓ 1 cup cooked chickpeas
- ✓ Three diced Roma tomatoes
- ✓ 3 tbsp Za'atar spice
- ✓ Salt to taste
- ✓ ½ chopped English cucumber
- ✓ 1 cup chopped parsley
- ✓ One chopped small red onion
- ✓ 1 cup chopped dill
- ✓ Garlic Vinaigrette
- ✓ Two chopped garlic cloves
- ✓ 1/3 cup extra virgin olive oil
- ✓ 2 tbsp lime juice
- ✓ Salt to taste
- ✓ Black pepper to taste

**Directions:**

- ❖ Season eggplant with salt and set aside for 30 minutes.
- ❖ Dry eggplant and cook in olive oil for five minutes from each side.
- ❖ When the eggplant has turned brown from both sides, remove the pan from the flame and keep it aside.
- ❖ In a bowl, combine cucumber, onions, tomatoes, dill, zaatar, chickpeas, parsley, and mix well.
- ❖ Place all the dressing ingredients in a bowl and toss well.
- ❖ Transfer cooked eggplant and chickpeas mixture in one large bowl and poured the dressing over them.
- ❖ Serve and enjoy it.

## 164) EASY ZUCCHINI SALAD WITH POMEGRANATE DRESSING

| Preparation Time: 8 minutes | Cooking Time: 15 minutes | Servings: 6 |
|---|---|---|

- ✓ One bunch of chives
- ✓ One pomegranate
- ✓ 1 tbsp pomegranate molasses
- ✓ 1/2 orange juice
- ✓ 1/4 cup mint leaf
- ✓ 120 g feta cheese
- ✓ 2 Lebanese cucumbers
- ✓ 2 tbsp currants
- ✓ 2 tbsp olive oil
- ✓ Three zucchinis
- ✓ salt and pepper

**Directions:**

- ❖ Clean the zucchini, then cucumber and slice the cucumber and cut it into ribbons using a peeler. And the same thing about your zucchini. Put the cucumber in the fridge.
- ❖ Chop chives into 2cm chunks and chop mint loosely.
- ❖ Make an orange Juice and combine with olive oil, a touch of pepper and salt, and 1 tbsp of pomegranate molasses to make the dressing. Whisk to blend.
- ❖ Toss the cucumber and zucchini into the dressing and apply the sliced herbs to prepare the salad.
- ❖ Add flowers and finish with the crumbled feta cheese.
- ❖ Slice the pomegranate into half and touch the skin's back with the dessert spoon to scatter the seeds over the salad.
- ❖ Now Serve.

## 165) ITALIAN-STYLE GRAIN SALAD

| Preparation Time: 5 minutes | Cooking Time: 35 minutes | Servings: 1 |
|---|---|---|

**Ingredients:**

- ✓ Coarse salt to taste
- ✓ Black pepper 2 tsp olive oil 1/2 minced small shallot 1/2 cup parsley, chopped 1
- ✓ 1 tbsp red wine vinegar 1 oz goat cheese, crumbled 1 cup grape tomatoes, halved

**Directions:**

- ❖ Combine the bulgur with 1/4 tsp salt and 1 cup of boiling water in a heat-proof dish. Cover, and let rest for about 30 minutes, before tender but somewhat chewy.
- ❖ Drain the bulgur and press to extract liquid in the fine-mesh sieve; return to the bowl. Add the onions, parsley, vinegar, shallot, and oil. Then season with pepper and salt, and toss.
- ❖ Top with cheese.

**Nutrition:** Calories:303 kcal Fat: 21g Protein: 10g Carbs: 21g Fiber: 4g

## 166) TROPICAL MACADAMIA NUTS DRESSING

| Preparation Time: 10 minutes | Cooking Time: 10 minutes | Servings: 4 |
|---|---|---|

**Ingredients:**

- ✓ ¼ tsp onion powder
- ✓ ½ tsp pepper
- ✓ 1 cup Cashew Milk
- ✓ 1 cup Macadamia Nuts
- ✓ 1 tbsp chives, chopped
- ✓ 1 tbsp lemon juice
- ✓ 1 tsp apple cider vinegar
- ✓ 1 tsp garlic powder
- ✓ 1 tsp salt
- ✓ 2 tbsp parsley

**Directions:**

- ❖ A high-powered mixer and places all the ingredients (other than green onions and chives, and parsley). Start at low and bring it up to high speed steadily until the ingredients are fully blended. If you want a thinner consistency, add more Homemade Cashew Milk from Nature's Eats.
- ❖ Add now the diced chives and parsley, then blend until smooth.
- ❖ Now serve promptly or store it in the refrigerator in an air-tight bag.

**Nutrition:** Calories: 302 kcal Fat: 26 g Protein: 8 g Carbs: 19 g Fiber: 6.3 g

## 167) EASY VINAIGRETTE DRESSING

| Preparation Time: 5 minutes | Cooking Time: 5 minutes | Servings: 1 |
|---|---|---|

- ✓ black pepper, to taste
- ✓ 3 tbsp vinegar
- ✓ Two cloves garlic, minced
- ✓ 1 tbsp honey
- ✓ 1 tbsp Dijon mustard
- ✓ ½ cup olive oil
- ✓ ¼ tsp salt

- ❖ Combine all the ingredients in a liquid mixing cup. With a small spoon or a fork, stir well till ingredients are thoroughly mixed together.
- ❖ Now taste, and customize as needed. Thin it out with a little more olive oil if the mixture becomes too acidic, or balance the flavors with a bit more maple, honey, or syrup. Add a pinch of salt if the mixture is a bit blah. If the zing is not enough, apply a tsp of vinegar.
- ❖ Serve instantly, or for potential use, cover, and refrigerate. For 7 to 10 days, the homemade vinaigrette lasts well. If the vinaigrette solidifies in the fridge somewhat, don't think about it. It helps to do this with real olive oil. Simply let it for 5 to 10 minutes at room temperature or microwave very quickly (approximately 20 secs) to liquefy that olive oil again. Now serve.

| 168) | Greek style turkey burger with Tzatziki sauce | |
|---|---|---|
| **Preparation Time:** 36 minutes | **Cooking Time:** 10 minutes | **Servings: 4** |

| Ingredients | | Directions |
|---|---|---|
| ✓ Turkey Burgers<br>✓ 1 lb ground turkey<br>✓ 1/3 cup chopped sun-dried tomatoes<br>✓ ½ cup chopped spinach leaves<br>✓ 1/4 cup chopped red onion<br>✓ 2 pressed garlic cloves<br>✓ ¼ cup feta cheese<br>✓ One egg<br>✓ 1 tsp dried oregano<br>✓ 1 tbsp olive oil<br>✓ 1/2 tsp kosher salt<br>✓ One sliced red onion | ✓ Four hamburger buns<br>✓ 1/2 tsp ground black pepper<br>✓ A handful of Bibb lettuce leaves<br>✓ Tzatziki Sauce<br>✓ ½ grated cucumber<br>✓ Two minced garlic cloves<br>✓ 3/4 cup Greek yogurt<br>✓ 1 tbsp red wine vinegar<br>✓ One pinch of kosher salt<br>✓ 1 tbsp chopped dill<br>✓ One pinch of black pepper | ❖ Combine all the ingredients of Tzatziki sauce in a bowl and mix well.<br>❖ Mix turkey, onion, sun-dried tomatoes, and feta cheese in a bowl.<br>❖ In another bowl, mix olive oil, egg, garlic, salt, oregano, and pepper.<br>❖ Pour egg mixture with turkey mixture. Mix well.<br>❖ Make medium-sized patties out of turkey mixture. Set aside in the refrigerator for 24 hours.<br>❖ Cook turkey patties on heated grill sprayed with oil for seven minutes from both sides on medium flame.<br>❖ Spread Tzatziki sauce over buns and place lettuce, onions, and cooked patties and serve. |

| 169) | SAUCY GREEK-STYLE BAKED SHRIMP | |
|---|---|---|
| **Preparation Time:** 15 minutes | **Cooking Time:** 20 minutes | **Servings: 4** |

| Ingredients | | Directions |
|---|---|---|
| ✓ 2 tbsp chopped dill<br>✓ 1 lb shrimp<br>✓ 1/4 tsp kosher salt<br>✓ 1/2 tsp red pepper flakes<br>✓ 3 tbsp olive oil<br>✓ Three minced garlic cloves | ✓ One chopped onion<br>✓ 15 oz crushed tomatoes<br>✓ 1/2 tsp ground cinnamon<br>✓ 1/2 tsp ground allspice<br>✓ 1/2 cup crumbled feta cheese | ❖ Add salt, shrimps, and pepper in a bowl. Toss well and keep it aside.<br>❖ Cook garlic and onions in heated olive oil over medium flame for five minutes.<br>❖ Add spices and stir for half a minute.<br>❖ Mix tomatoes and let it simmer for 20 minutes with occasional stirring.<br>❖ Transfer the tomato mixture to the baking sheet and add shrimps to it. Spread cheese and bake in a preheated oven at 375 degrees for 20 minutes.<br>❖ Drizzle dill and serve. |

| 170) | TASTY SAUTÉED CHICKEN WITH OLIVES CAPERS AND LEMONS | |
|---|---|---|
| **Preparation Time:** 5 minutes | **Cooking Time:** 30 minutes | **Servings: 4** |

| Ingredients | | Directions |
|---|---|---|
| ✓ Six boneless chicken thighs<br>✓ Two sliced lemons<br>✓ One minced garlic clove minced<br>✓ 2/4 cup extra virgin olive oil<br>✓ 2 tbsp all-purpose flour | ✓ 2 tbsp butter<br>✓ 1 cup chicken broth<br>✓ kosher salt to taste<br>✓ 3/4 cup Sicilian green olives<br>✓ 2 tbsp parsley<br>✓ 1/4 cup capers<br>✓ Black pepper to taste | ❖ Add salt, chicken, and pepper in a bowl and toss well. Set aside for 15 minutes.<br>❖ Cook lemon slices (half of them) in heated olive oil over medium flame for five minutes from both sides.<br>❖ Shift the cooked brown lemon slices on the plate.<br>❖ Coat chicken pieces with rice flour and cook in heated olive oil in the skillet for seven minutes from both sides. Transfer the cooked chicken to the plate.<br>❖ Sauté garlic in heated oil in the same pan for about half a minute. Stir in olives, chicken broth, lemons, and capers. Cook over high flame for few minutes.<br>❖ When half of the broth is left, add parsley and butter. Cook for one minute.<br>❖ Add salt and pepper to adjust the taste and serve. |

## 171)   ENGLISH PORRIDGE (OATMEAL)

| Preparation Time: 2 minutes | Cooking Time: 2 minutes | Servings: 1 |
|---|---|---|

**Ingredients:**

- ✓ Base Recipe
- ✓ ½ cup oats
- ✓ 1/2cup water
- ✓ 1/2cup milk
- ✓ 1 Pinch salt
- ✓ Maple Brown Sugar
- ✓ 1 tsp sugar
- ✓ 2 tbsp chopped pecans
- ✓ 1 tsp maple syrup
- ✓ 1/8 tsp cinnamon
- ✓ Banana Nut
- ✓ ½ banana sliced
- ✓ 1 tbsp flaxseed
- ✓ 2 tbsp walnuts
- ✓ 1/8 tsp cinnamon
- ✓ Strawberry & Cream
- ✓ 1/2cup strawberries
- ✓ 2 tsp honey
- ✓ 1 tbsp half and half
- ✓ 1/8 tsp vanilla extract
- ✓ Chocolate Peanut Butter
- ✓ 2 tsp cocoa powder
- ✓ 2 tsp chocolate chips
- ✓ 1 tbsp peanut butter
- ✓ 1 tsp roasted peanuts

**Directions:**

- ❖ Microwave Instructions
- ❖ Place all the ingredients heat in the microwave on high for 2 minutes. Then add 15-sec increments until the oatmeal is puffed and softened.
- ❖ Stovetop Instructions
- ❖ Bring the water and milk to a boil in a pan. Lower the heat & pour in the oats. Cook it while stirring, till the oats are soft and have absorbed most of the liquid.Turn off the stove and let it for 2 to 3 min.
- ❖ Assembly
- ❖ Stir in the toppings and let rest for a few minutes to cool. Serve warm.

**Nutrition:** Calories: 227 kcal Fat:6 g Protein: 9 g Carbs: 33 g Fiber: 4 g

## 172)   MOROCCAN SALAD FATTOUSH

| Preparation Time: 20 minutes | Cooking Time: 20 minutes | Servings: 6 |
|---|---|---|

**Ingredients:**

- ✓ Two loaves of pita bread
- ✓ • ½ tsp sumac
- ✓ • Olive Oil
- ✓ • Salt and pepper
- ✓ • One chopped English cucumber
- ✓ • One chopped lettuce
- ✓ • Five chopped Roma tomatoes
- ✓ Five radishes
- ✓ • Five chopped green onions
- ✓ • 2 cup parsley leaves
- ✓ Lime-vinaigrette
- ✓ • 1/4 tsp cinnamon
- ✓ • 1 tsp lime juice
- ✓ • Salt and pepper
- ✓ • 1/3 cup Virgin Olive Oil
- ✓ • 1 tsp sumac
- ✓ • 1/4 tsp allspice

**Directions:**

- ❖ Toast the bread in the oven. Heat olive oil and fry until browned. Add salt, pepper, and 1/2tsp of sumac. Turn off heat & place pita chips on paper towels to drain.
- ❖ In a mixing bowl, mix the chopped lettuce, cucumber, tomatoes, green onions with the sliced radish and parsley.
- ❖ For seasoning, whisk the lemon or lime juice, olive oil, and spices in a small bowl.
- ❖ Sprinkle the salad & toss lightly. Finally, add the pita chips and more sumac if you like. Shifts to small serving bowls or plates. Enjoy!

**Nutrition:** Calories: 345 kcal Fat:20.4 g Protein: 9.1 g Carbs:39.8 g Fiber: 1 g

## 173) CALABRIA CICORIA E FAGIOLI

| Preparation Time: | Cooking Time: | Servings: 6 |
|---|---|---|

| Ingredients: | | Directions: |
|---|---|---|
| ✓ 200 g dried cannellini beans<br>✓ • 6 tbsp olive oil<br>✓ • 400 g curly endive | ✓ Four garlic cloves<br>✓ • 600 ml of water<br>✓ • Two red chilies<br>✓ • Salt and pepper to taste | ❖ Put the dried beans to soak for 12 h (they increase in size). Drain them and boil for two h in fresh unsalted water. Salt at the end of the cooking time. If using canned beans, drain them from their liquid and rinse them before use. Rinse the endive and cut it up into short lengths.<br><br>❖ Heat the olive oil, fry the garlic without browning, and then add the endive and chilies. Keeping the heat high, stir-fry for a minute or two, coating the endive with the oil, then add the drained cannellini beans, some salt, and the water. Bring to the boil, cover the pan, and lower the heat. Cook until the endive is soft and most of the liquid has been absorbed. |

**Nutrition:** Calories:225 kcal Fat: 21 g Protein: 3 g Carbs: 6 g Fiber:1 g

## 174) CAMPANIA POACHED EGGS CAPRESE

| Preparation Time: 10 minutes | Cooking Time: 10 minutes | Servings: 2 |
|---|---|---|

| Ingredients: | | Directions: |
|---|---|---|
| ✓ 4 tsp pesto<br>✓ • 1 tbsp white vinegar<br>✓ • Four eggs<br>✓ • 2 tsp salt | ✓ 2 English muffins<br>✓ • salt to taste<br>✓ • One tomato sliced<br>✓ • Four slices of mozzarella cheese | ❖ Fill 2 to 3 inches of a pan with water and boil over a high flame. Lower the heat, add the vinegar, 2 tsp of salt in it, and let it simmer.<br><br>❖ Put a cheese slice and a slice of tomato on every English muffin half and put in a toaster oven for 5 min or till the cheese melts and the English muffin is well toasted.<br><br>❖ Break an egg in a bowl and add in the water one by one. Let the eggs cook for 2.5 to 3 minutes or until the yolks have solidified and the egg whites are firm. Take the eggs out of the water and put them on a kitchen towel to absorb excess water.<br><br>❖ For assembling, first put an egg on top of every muffin, add a tsp of pesto sauce on the egg, and scatter the salt. |

## 175) GREEK BREAKFAST DISH WITH EGGS AND VEGETABLES

| Preparation Time: 10 minutes | Cooking Time: 10 minutes | Servings: 2 |
|---|---|---|

| Ingredients: | | Directions: |
|---|---|---|
| ✓ 1 tbsp olive oil<br>✓ • salt to taste<br>✓ • 2 cup chopped rainbow chard<br>✓ • ½ cup arugula | ✓ 1 cup spinach<br>✓ • Two cloves garlic<br>✓ • ½ cup grated Cheddar cheese<br>✓ • Four eggs<br>✓ • black pepper to taste | ❖ Heat oil over moderate pressure. Sauté the chard, spinach, and arugula until soft, around three minutes. Add garlic, continue cooking until aromatic, approx. Two min.<br><br>❖ In a cup, combine the eggs and the cheese; dump into the mixture of the chard. Heat and cook for 5 - 6 minutes. Season to taste with salt and pepper. |

## 176) ITALIAN BREAKFAST PITA PIZZA

| Preparation Time: 25 minutes | Cooking Time: 30 minutes | Servings: 2 |
|---|---|---|

**Ingredients:**

- ✓ Four slices of bacon
- ✓ 2 tbsp olive oil
- ✓ 1/4 onion
- ✓ Four eggs
- ✓ Two pita bread rounds
- ✓ 2 tbsp pesto
- ✓ ½ tomato
- ✓ One avocado
- ✓ ½ cup slashed spinach
- ✓ 1/4 cup mushrooms
- ✓ ½ cup grated Cheddar cheese

**Directions:**

- ❖ Heat the oven to 350 ° F (175° C).
- ❖ In a medium saucepan, put the bacon and cook over medium-high heat, rotating periodically, when browned uniformly, around ten minutes. Cook the onion in the same skillet till smooth. Put it aside. In the skillet, melt the olive oil. Add the eggs and cook, stirring regularly, for 3 to 5 minutes.
- ❖ Add the pita bread to the cake pan. Cover with bacon, fried eggs, onions, mushrooms, and spinach; sprinkle the pesto over through the pita. Dress over the toppings of Cheddar cheese.
- ❖ Bake it in the preheated oven for10 min. Serve with avocado pieces.

## 177) NAPOLI CAPRESE ON TOAST

| Preparation Time: 15 minutes | Cooking Time: 5 minutes | Servings: 14 |
|---|---|---|

- ✓ 14 slices bread
- ✓ 1 lb mozzarella cheese
- ✓ Two cloves garlic
- ✓ 1/3 cup basil leaves
- ✓ 3 tbsp olive oil
- ✓ Three tomatoes
- ✓ salt to taste
- ✓ black pepper to taste

**Directions:**

- ❖ Baked the bread slices and spread the garlic on one side of each piece. Put a slice of mozzarella cheese, 1 to 2 basil leaves, and a slice of tomato on each piece of toast. Sprinkle with olive oil, spray salt, and black pepper.

**Nutrition:** Calories: 203.5 kcal Fat: 10 g Protein: 10.5 g Carbs: 16.5 g Fiber: 1.1 g

## 178) TUSCAN EGGS FLORENTINE

| Preparation Time: 10 minutes | Cooking Time: 10 minutes | Servings: 3 |
|---|---|---|

**Ingredients:**

- ✓ 2 tbsp butter
- ✓ Two cloves garlic
- ✓ 3 tbsp cream cheese
- ✓ ½ cup mushroom
- ✓ ½ fresh spinach
- ✓ Salt to taste
- ✓ Six eggs
- ✓ Black pepper to taste

**Directions:**

- ❖ Put the butter in a non-stick skillet; heat and mix the mushrooms and garlic till the garlic is flavorsome for about 1 min. Add spinach to the mushroom paste and cook until spinach is softened for 2 - 3 mins,
- ❖ Mix the mushroom-spinach mixer; add salt and pepper. Cook, with mixing, until the eggs are stiff; turn. Pour with cream cheese over the egg mixture and cook before cream cheese started melting just over five minutes.

**Nutrition:** Calories: 278.9 kcal Fat: 22.9 g Protein:15.7 g Carbs: 4.1 g Fiber:22.9

## 179) SPECIAL QUINOA, CEREALS FOR BREAKFAST

| Preparation Time: 5 minutes | Cooking Time: 16 minutes | Servings: 4 |
|---|---|---|

**Ingredients:**

- ✓ 2 cups of water
- ✓ ½ cup apricots
- ✓ 1 cup quinoa
- ✓ ½ cup almonds
- ✓ 1 tsp cinnamon
- ✓ 1/3 cup seeds
- ✓ ½ tsp nutmeg

**Directions:**

- ❖ Combine water and quinoa in a medium saucepan and continue cooking. Lower the heat and boil when much of the water has been drained for 8–12 minutes. Whisk in apricots, almonds, linseeds, cinnamon, and nutmeg; simmer till the quinoa is soft.

**Nutrition:** Calories: 349.9 kcal Fat:15.1 g Protein: 11.8 g Carbs: 44.5 g Fiber: 9.3 g

## 180) SIMPLE ZUCCHINI WITH EGG

| Preparation Time: 5 minutes | Cooking Time: 15 minutes | Servings: 2 |
|---|---|---|

**Ingredients:**

- ✓ Two eggs
- ✓ 1.5 tbsp olive oil
- ✓ salt to taste
- ✓ Two zucchinis
- ✓ Black pepper to taste
- ✓ 1 tsp water

**Directions:**

- ❖ Heat the oil in a saucepan over medium heat; sauté the zucchini until soft, around 10 minutes. Season with salt and black pepper.
- ❖ Add the eggs with a fork in a bowl; add more water and mix until uniformly mixed. Spill the eggs over the zucchini; continue cooking until the eggs are boiled and rubbery for almost 5 minutes. Dress it with salt and black pepper.

**Nutrition:** Calories: 21.7 kcal Fat: 15.7 g Protein: 10.2 g Carbs: 11.2 g Fiber: 3.6 g

## 181) ITALIAN BAKED EGGS IN AVOCADO

| Preparation Time: 10 minutes | Cooking Time: 15 minutes | Servings: 2 |
|---|---|---|

- ✓ One pinch parsley
- ✓ Two eggs
- ✓ Two slice bacon
- ✓ One avocado
- ✓ 2 tsp chives
- ✓ One pinch of salt and black pepper

- ❖ Preheat the oven to 425 degrees.
- ❖ Break the eggs in a tub, willing to maintain the yolks preserved.
- ❖ Assemble the avocado halves in the baking bowl, rest them on the side. Slowly spoon one egg yolk in the avocado opening. Keep spooning the white egg into the hole till it is finished. Do the same with leftover egg yolk, egg white, and avocado. Dress with chives, parsley, sea salt, and pepper for each of the avocados.
- ❖ Gently put the baking dish in the preheated oven and cook for about 15 min well before the eggs are cooked. Sprinkle with bacon over the avocado.

## 182) SPECIAL GROUND PORK SKILLET

| | Cooking Time: 25 Minutes | Servings: 4 |
|---|---|---|

- ✓ 1 ½ pounds ground pork
- ✓ 2 tbsp olive oil
- ✓ 1 bunch kale, trimmed and roughly chopped
- ✓ 1 cup onions, sliced
- ✓ 1/4 tsp black pepper, or more to taste
- ✓ 1/4 cup tomato puree
- ✓ 1 bell pepper, chopped
- ✓ 1 tsp sea salt
- ✓ 1 cup chicken bone broth
- ✓ 1/4 cup port wine
- ✓ 2 cloves garlic, pressed
- ✓ 1 chili pepper, sliced

- ❖ Heat tbsp of the olive oil in a cast-iron skillet over a moderately high heat. Now, sauté the onion, garlic, and peppers until they are tender and fragrant; reserve.
- ❖ Heat the remaining tbsp of olive oil; once hot, cook the ground pork and approximately 5 minutes until no longer pink.
- ❖ Add in the other ingredients and continue to cook for 15 to 17 minutes or until cooked through.
- ❖ Storing
- ❖ Place the ground pork mixture in airtight containers or Ziploc bags; keep in your refrigerator for up to 3 to 4 days.
- ❖ For freezing, place the ground pork mixture in airtight containers or heavy-duty freezer bags. Freeze up to 2 to 3 months. Defrost in the refrigerator. Bon appétit!

**Nutrition:** 349 Calories; 13g Fat; 4.4g Carbs; 45.3g Protein; 1.2g Fiber

## 183) DELICIOUS GREEK STYLE CHEESE PORK

| Cooking Time: 20 Minutes | Servings: 6 |
|---|---|

| | | |
|---|---|---|
| ✓ 1 tbsp sesame oil<br>✓ 1 ½ pounds pork shoulder, cut into strips<br>✓ Himalayan salt and freshly ground black pepper, to taste<br>✓ 1/2 tsp cayenne pepper<br>✓ 1/2 cup shallots, roughly chopped | ✓ 2 bell peppers, sliced<br>✓ 1/4 cup cream of onion soup<br>✓ 1/2 tsp Sriracha sauce<br>✓ 1 tbsp tahini (sesame butter<br>✓ 1 tbsp soy sauce<br>✓ 4 ounces gouda cheese, cut into small pieces | ❖ Heat he sesame oil in a wok over a moderately high flame.<br>❖ Stir-fry the pork strips for 3 to 4 minutes or until just browned on all sides. Add in the spices, shallots and bell peppers and continue to cook for a further 4 minutes.<br>❖ Stir in the cream of onion soup, Sriracha, sesame butter, and soy sauce; continue to cook for to 4 minutes more.<br>❖ Top with the cheese and continue to cook until the cheese has melted.<br>❖ Storing<br>❖ Place your stir-fry in six airtight containers or Ziploc bags; keep in your refrigerator for 3 to 4 days.<br>❖ For freezing, wrap tightly with heavy-duty aluminum foil or freezer wrap. It will maintain the best quality for 2 to 3 months. Defrost in the refrigerator and reheat in your wok. |

**Nutrition:** 424 Calories; 29.4g Fat; 3. Carbs; 34.2g Protein; 0.6g Fiber

## 184) SPECIAL PORK IN BLUE CHEESE SAUCE

| Cooking Time: 30 Minutes | Servings: 6 |
|---|---|

| | | |
|---|---|---|
| ✓ 2 pounds pork center cut loin roast, boneless and cut into 6 pieces<br>✓ 1 tbsp coconut aminos<br>✓ 6 ounces blue cheese<br>✓ 1/3 cup heavy cream<br>✓ 1/3 cup port wine | ✓ 1/3 cup roasted vegetable broth, preferably homemade<br>✓ 1 tsp dried hot chile flakes<br>✓ 1 tsp dried rosemary<br>✓ 1 tbsp lard<br>✓ 1 shallot, chopped<br>✓ 2 garlic cloves, chopped<br>✓ Salt and freshly cracked black peppercorns, to taste | ❖ Rub each piece of the pork with salt, black peppercorns, and rosemary.<br>❖ Melt the lard in a saucepan over a moderately high flame. Sear the pork on all sides about 15 minutes; set aside.<br>❖ Cook the shallot and garlic until they've softened. Add in port wine to scrape up any brown bits from the bottom.<br>❖ Reduce the heat to medium-low and add in the remaining ingredients; continue to simmer until the sauce has thickened and reduced.<br>❖ Storing<br>❖ Divide the pork and sauce into six portions; place each portion in a separate airtight container or Ziploc bag; keep in your refrigerator for 3 to 4 days.<br>❖ Freeze the pork and sauce in airtight containers or heavy-duty freezer bags. Freeze up to 4 months. Defrost in the refrigerator. Bon appétit! |

## 185) MISSISSIPPI-STYLE PULLED PORK

| Cooking Time: 6 Hours | Servings: 4 |
|---|---|

| | | |
|---|---|---|
| ✓ 1 ½ pounds pork shoulder<br>✓ 1 tbsp liquid smoke sauce<br>✓ 1 tsp chipotle powder | ✓ Au Jus gravy seasoning packet<br>✓ 2 onions, cut into wedges<br>✓ Kosher salt and freshly ground black pepper, taste | ❖ Mix the liquid smoke sauce, chipotle powder, Au Jus gravy seasoning packet, salt and pepper. Rub the spice mixture into the pork on all sides.<br>❖ Wrap in plastic wrap and let it marinate in your refrigerator for 3 hours.<br>❖ Prepare your grill for indirect heat. Place the pork butt roast on the grate over a drip pan and top with onions; cover the grill and cook for about 6 hours.<br>❖ Transfer the pork to a cutting board. Now, shred the meat into bite-sized pieces using two forks.<br>❖ Storing<br>❖ Divide the pork between four airtight containers or Ziploc bags; keep in your refrigerator for up to 3 to 5 days.<br>❖ For freezing, place the pork in airtight containers or heavy-duty freezer bags. Freeze up to 4 months. Defrost in the refrigerator. Bon appétit! |

## 186) SPICY WITH CHEESY TURKEY DIP

| | Cooking Time: 25 Minutes | Servings: 4 |
|---|---|---|

| Ingredients | | Instructions |
|---|---|---|
| ✓ 1 Fresno chili pepper, deveined and minced<br>✓ 1 ½ cups Ricotta cheese, creamed, 4% fat, softened<br>✓ 1/4 cup sour cream<br>✓ 1 tbsp butter, room temperature<br>✓ 1 shallot, chopped | ✓ 1 tsp garlic, pressed<br>✓ 1 pound ground turkey<br>✓ 1/2 cup goat cheese, shredded<br>✓ Salt and black pepper, to taste<br>✓ 1 ½ cups Gruyère, shredded | ❖ Melt the butter in a frying pan over a moderately high flame. Now, sauté the onion and garlic until they have softened.<br>❖ Stir in the ground turkey and continue to cook until it is no longer pink.<br>❖ Transfer the sautéed mixture to a lightly greased baking dish. Add in Ricotta, sour cream, goat cheese, salt, pepper, and chili pepper.<br>❖ Top with the shredded Gruyère cheese. Bake in the preheated oven at 350 degrees F for about 20 minutes or until hot and bubbly in top.<br>❖ Storing<br>❖ Place your dip in an airtight container; keep in your refrigerator for up 3 to 4 days. Enjoy! |

**Nutrition:** 284 Calories; 19g Fat; 3.2g Carbs; 26. Protein; 1.6g Fiber

## 187) TURKEY CHORIZO AND BOK CHOY

| | Cooking Time: 50 Minutes | Servings: 4 |
|---|---|---|

| Ingredients | | Instructions |
|---|---|---|
| ✓ 4 mild turkey Chorizo, sliced<br>✓ 1/2 cup full-fat milk<br>✓ 6 ounces Gruyère cheese, preferably freshly grated<br>✓ 1 yellow onion, chopped | Coarse salt and ground black pepper, to taste<br>✓ 1 pound Bok choy, tough stem ends trimmed<br>✓ 1 cup cream of mushroom soup<br>✓ 1 tbsp lard, room temperature | ❖ Melt the lard in a nonstick skillet over a moderate flame; cook the Chorizo sausage for about 5 minutes, stirring occasionally to ensure even cooking; reserve.<br>❖ Add in the onion, salt, pepper, Bok choy, and cream of mushroom soup. Continue to cook for 4 minutes longer or until the vegetables have softened.<br>❖ Spoon the mixture into a lightly oiled casserole dish. Top with the reserved Chorizo.<br>❖ In a mixing bowl, thoroughly combine the milk and cheese. Pour the cheese mixture over the sausage.<br>❖ Cover with foil and bake at 36degrees F for about 35 minutes.<br>❖ Storing<br>❖ Cut your casserole into four portions. Place each portion in an airtight container; keep in your refrigerator for 3 to 4 days.<br>❖ For freezing, wrap your portions tightly with heavy-duty aluminum foil or freezer wrap. Freeze up to 1 to 2 months. Defrost in the refrigerator. Enjoy! |

## 188) CLASSIC SPICY CHICKEN BREASTS

| | Cooking Time: 30 Minutes | Servings: 6 |
|---|---|---|

| Ingredients | | Instructions |
|---|---|---|
| ✓ 1 ½ pounds chicken breasts<br>✓ 1 bell pepper, deveined and chopped<br>✓ 1 leek, chopped<br>✓ 1 tomato, pureed<br>✓ 2 tbsp coriander | ✓ 2 garlic cloves, minced<br>✓ 1 tsp cayenne pepper<br>✓ 1 tsp dry thyme<br>✓ 1/4 cup coconut aminos<br>✓ Sea salt and ground black pepper, to taste | ❖ Rub each chicken breasts with the garlic, cayenne pepper, thyme, salt and black pepper. Cook the chicken in a saucepan over medium-high heat.<br>❖ Sear for about 5 minutes until golden brown on all sides.<br>❖ Fold in the tomato puree and coconut aminos and bring it to a boil. Add in the pepper, leek, and coriander.<br>❖ Reduce the heat to simmer. Continue to cook, partially covered, for about 20 minutes.<br>❖ Storing<br>❖ Place the chicken breasts in airtight containers or Ziploc bags; keep in your refrigerator for 3 to 4 days.<br>❖ For freezing, place the chicken breasts in airtight containers or heavy-duty freezer bags. It will maintain the best quality for about 4 months. Defrost in the refrigerator. Bon appétit! |

## 189) DELICIOUS SAUCY BOSTON BUTT

| | Cooking Time: 1 Hour 20 Minutes | Servings: 8 |
|---|---|---|

| | | |
|---|---|---|
| ✓ 1 tbsp lard, room temperature<br>✓ 2 pounds Boston butt, cubed<br>✓ Salt and freshly ground pepper<br>✓ 1/2 tsp mustard powder<br>✓ A bunch of spring onions, chopped | ✓ 2 garlic cloves, minced<br>✓ 1/2 tbsp ground cardamom<br>✓ 2 tomatoes, pureed<br>✓ 1 bell pepper, deveined and chopped<br>✓ 1 jalapeno pepper, deveined and finely chopped<br>✓ 1/2 cup unsweetened coconut milk<br>✓ 2 cups chicken bone broth | ❖ In a wok, melt the lard over moderate heat. Season the pork belly with salt, pepper and mustard powder.<br>❖ Sear the pork for 8 to 10 minutes, stirring periodically to ensure even cooking; set aside, keeping it warm.<br>❖ In the same wok, sauté the spring onions, garlic, and cardamom. Spoon the sautéed vegetables along with the reserved pork into the slow cooker.<br>❖ Add in the remaining ingredients, cover with the lid and cook for 1 hour 10 minutes over low heat.<br>❖ Divide the pork and vegetables between airtight containers or Ziploc bags; keep in your refrigerator for up to 3 to 5 days.<br>❖ For freezing, place the pork and vegetables in airtight containers or heavy-duty freezer bags. Freeze up to 4 months. Defrost in the refrigerator. Bon appétit! |

## 190) SPECIAL OLD-FASHIONED HUNGARIAN GOULASH

| | Cooking Time: 9 Hours 10 Minutes | Servings: 4 |
|---|---|---|

| | | |
|---|---|---|
| ✓ 1 ½ pounds pork butt, chopped<br>✓ 1 tsp sweet Hungarian paprika<br>✓ 2 Hungarian hot peppers, deveined and minced<br>✓ 1 cup leeks, chopped<br>✓ 1 ½ tbsp lard<br>✓ 1 tsp caraway seeds, ground<br>✓ 4 cups vegetable broth<br>✓ 2 garlic cloves, crushed<br>✓ 1 tsp cayenne pepper<br>✓ 2 cups tomato sauce with herbs | ✓ 1 ½ pounds pork butt, chopped<br>✓ 1 tsp sweet Hungarian paprika<br>✓ 2 Hungarian hot peppers, deveined and minced<br>✓ 1 cup leeks, chopped<br>✓ 1 ½ tbsp lard<br>✓ 1 tsp caraway seeds, ground<br>✓ 4 cups vegetable broth<br>✓ 2 garlic cloves, crushed<br>✓ 1 tsp cayenne pepper<br>✓ 2 cups tomato sauce with herbs | ❖ Melt the lard in a heavy-bottomed pot over medium-high heat. Sear the pork for 5 to 6 minutes until just browned on all sides; set aside.<br>❖ Add in the leeks and garlic; continue to cook until they have softened.<br>❖ Place the reserved pork along with the sautéed mixture in your crock pot. Add in the other ingredients and stir to combine.<br>❖ Cover with the lid and slow cook for 9 hours on the lowest setting.<br>❖ Storing<br>❖ Spoon your goulash into four airtight containers or Ziploc bags; keep in your refrigerator for up to 3 to 4 days.<br>❖ For freezing, place the goulash in airtight containers. Freeze up to 4 to 6 months. Defrost in the refrigerator. Enjoy! |

## 191) TYPICAL ITALIAN-STYLE CHEESY PORK LOIN

| | Cooking Time: 25 Minutes | Servings: 4 |
|---|---|---|

| | | |
|---|---|---|
| ✓ 1 pound pork loin, cut into 1-inch-thick pieces<br>✓ 1 tsp Italian seasoning mix<br>✓ Salt and pepper, to taste<br>✓ 1 onion, sliced<br>✓ 1 tsp fresh garlic, smashed<br>✓ 2 tbsp black olives, pitted and sliced | ✓ 2 tbsp balsamic vinegar<br>✓ 1/2 cup Romano cheese, grated<br>✓ 2 tbsp butter, room temperature<br>✓ 1 tbsp curry paste<br>✓ 1 cup roasted vegetable broth<br>✓ 1 tbsp oyster sauce | ❖ In a frying pan, melt the butter over a moderately high heat. Once hot, cook the pork until browned on all sides; season with salt and black pepper and set aside.<br>❖ In the pan drippings, cook the onion and garlic for 4 to 5 minutes or until they've softened.<br>❖ Add in the Italian seasoning mix, curry paste, and vegetable broth. Continue to cook until the sauce has thickened and reduced slightly or about 10 minutes. Add in the remaining ingredients along with the reserved pork.<br>❖ Top with cheese and cook for 10 minutes longer or until cooked through.<br>❖ Storing<br>❖ Divide the pork loin between four airtight containers; keep in your refrigerator for 3 to 5 days.<br>❖ For freezing, place the pork loin in airtight containers or heavy-duty freezer bags. Freeze up to 4 to 6 months. Defrost in the refrigerator. Enjoy! |

## 192) BAKED SPARE RIBS

| | Cooking Time: 3 Hour 40 Minutes | Servings: 6 |
|---|---|---|

**Ingredients:**

- ✓ 2 pounds spare ribs
- ✓ 1 garlic clove, minced
- ✓ 1 tsp dried marjoram
- ✓ 1 lime, halved
- ✓ Salt and ground black pepper, to taste

**Directions:**

- ❖ Toss all ingredients in a ceramic dish.
- ❖ Cover and let it refrigerate for 5 to 6 hours.
- ❖ Roast the foil-wrapped ribs in the preheated oven at 275 degrees F degrees for about hours 30 minutes.
- ❖ Storing
- ❖ Divide the ribs into six portions. Place each portion of ribs in an airtight container; keep in your refrigerator for 3 to days.
- ❖ For freezing, place the ribs in airtight containers or heavy-duty freezer bags. Freeze up to 4 to months. Defrost in the refrigerator and reheat in the preheated oven. Bon appétit!

## 193) HEALTHY CHICKEN PARMESAN SALAD

| | Cooking Time: 20 Minutes | Servings: 6 |
|---|---|---|

- ✓ 2 romaine hearts, leaves separated
- ✓ Flaky sea salt and ground black pepper, to taste
- ✓ 1/4 tsp chili pepper flakes
- ✓ 1 tsp dried basil
- ✓ 1/4 cup Parmesan, finely grated
- ✓ 2 chicken breasts
- ✓ 2 Lebanese cucumbers, sliced
- ✓ For the dressing:
- ✓ 2 large egg yolks
- ✓ 1 tsp Dijon mustard
- ✓ 1 tbsp fresh lemon juice
- ✓ 1/4 cup olive oil
- ✓ 2 garlic cloves, minced

**Directions:**

- ❖ In a grilling pan, cook the chicken breast until no longer pink or until a meat thermometer registers 5 degrees F. Slice the chicken into strips.
- ❖ Storing
- ❖ Place the chicken breasts in airtight containers or Ziploc bags; keep in your refrigerator for to 4 days.
- ❖ For freezing, place the chicken breasts in airtight containers or heavy-duty freezer bags. It will maintain the best quality for about months. Defrost in the refrigerator.
- ❖ Toss the chicken with the other ingredients. Prepare the dressing by whisking all the ingredients.
- ❖ Dress the salad and enjoy! Keep the salad in your refrigerator for 3 to 5 days.

## 194) CLASSIC TURKEY WINGS WITH GRAVY SAUCE

| | Cooking Time: 6 Hours | Servings: 6 |
|---|---|---|

**Ingredients:**

- ✓ 2 pounds turkey wings
- ✓ 1/2 tsp cayenne pepper
- ✓ 4 garlic cloves, sliced
- ✓ 1 large onion, chopped
- ✓ Salt and pepper, to taste
- ✓ 1 tsp dried marjoram
- ✓ 1 tbsp butter, room temperature
- ✓ 1 tbsp Dijon mustard
- ✓ For the Gravy:
- ✓ 1 cup double cream
- ✓ Salt and black pepper, to taste
- ✓ 1/2 stick butter
- ✓ 3/4 tsp guar gum

**Directions:**

- ❖ Rub the turkey wings with the Dijon mustard and tbsp of butter. Preheat a grill pan over medium-high heat.
- ❖ Sear the turkey wings for 10 minutes on all sides.
- ❖ Transfer the turkey to your Crock pot; add in the garlic, onion, salt, pepper, marjoram, and cayenne pepper. Cover and cook on low setting for 6 hours.
- ❖ Melt 1/2 stick of the butter in a frying pan. Add in the cream and whisk until cooked through.
- ❖ Next, stir in the guar gum, salt, and black pepper along with cooking juices. Let it cook until the sauce has reduced by half.
- ❖ Storing
- ❖ Wrap the turkey wings in foil before packing them into airtight containers; keep in your refrigerator for up to 3 to 4 days.
- ❖ For freezing, place the turkey wings in airtight containers or heavy-duty freezer bags. Freeze up to 2 to 3 months. Defrost in the refrigerator.
- ❖ Keep your gravy in refrigerator for up to 2 days.

## 195) AUTHENTIC PORK CHOPS WITH HERBS

| | Cooking Time: 20 Minutes | Servings: 4 |
|---|---|---|

**Ingredients:**

- ✓ 1 tbsp butter
- ✓ 1 pound pork chops
- ✓ 2 rosemary sprigs, minced
- ✓ 1 tsp dried marjoram
- ✓ 1 tsp dried parsley
- ✓ A bunch of spring onions, roughly chopped
- ✓ 1 thyme sprig, minced
- ✓ 1/2 tsp granulated garlic
- ✓ 1/2 tsp paprika, crushed
- ✓ Coarse salt and ground black pepper, to taste

- ❖ Season the pork chops with the granulated garlic, paprika, salt, and black pepper.
- ❖ Melt the butter in a frying pan over a moderate flame. Cook the pork chops for 6 to 8 minutes, turning them occasionally to ensure even cooking.
- ❖ Add in the remaining ingredients and cook an additional 4 minutes.
- ❖ Storing
- ❖ Divide the pork chops into four portions; place each portion in a separate airtight container or Ziploc bag; keep in your refrigerator for 3 to 4 days.
- ❖ Freeze the pork chops in airtight containers or heavy-duty freezer bags. Freeze up to 4 months. Defrost in the refrigerator. Bon appétit!

## 196) PEPPERS STUFFED WITH CHOPPED PORK ORIGINAL

| | Cooking Time: 40 Minutes | Servings: 4 |
|---|---|---|

**Ingredients:**

- ✓ 6 bell peppers, deveined
- ✓ 1 tbsp vegetable oil
- ✓ 1 shallot, chopped
- ✓ 1 garlic clove, minced
- ✓ 1/2 pound ground pork
- ✓ 1/3 pound ground veal
- ✓ 1 ripe tomato, chopped
- ✓ 1/2 tsp mustard seeds
- ✓ Sea salt and ground black pepper, to taste

- ❖ Parboil the peppers for 5 minutes.
- ❖ Heat the vegetable oil in a frying pan that is preheated over a moderate heat. Cook the shallot and garlic for 3 to 4 minutes until they've softened.
- ❖ Stir in the ground meat and cook, breaking apart with a fork, for about 6 minutes. Add the chopped tomatoes, mustard seeds, salt, and pepper.
- ❖ Continue to cook for 5 minutes or until heated through. Divide the filling between the peppers and transfer them to a baking pan.
- ❖ Bake in the preheated oven at 36degrees F approximately 25 minutes.
- ❖ Storing
- ❖ Place the peppers in airtight containers or Ziploc bags; keep in your refrigerator for up to 3 to 4 days.
- ❖ For freezing, place the peppers in airtight containers or heavy-duty freezer bags. Freeze up to 2 to 3 months. Defrost in the refrigerator. Bon appétit!

**Nutrition:** 2 Calories; 20.5g Fat; 8.2g Carbs; 18.2g Protein; 1.5g Fiber

## 197) GRILL-STYLE CHICKEN SALAD WITH AVOCADO

| Cooking Time: 20 Minutes | Servings: 4 |
|---|---|

**Ingredients:**

- ✓ 1/3 cup olive oil
- ✓ 2 chicken breasts
- ✓ Sea salt and crushed red pepper flakes
- ✓ 2 egg yolks
- ✓ 1 tbsp fresh lemon juice
- ✓ 1/2 tsp celery seeds
- ✓ 1 tbsp coconut aminos
- ✓ 1 large-sized avocado, pitted and sliced

**Directions:**

- ❖ Grill the chicken breasts for about 4 minutes per side. Season with salt and pepper, to taste.
- ❖ Slice the grilled chicken into bite-sized strips.
- ❖ To make the dressing, whisk the egg yolks, lemon juice, celery seeds, olive oil and coconut aminos in a measuring cup.
- ❖ Storing
- ❖ Place the chicken breasts in airtight containers or Ziploc bags; keep in your refrigerator for 3 to 4 days.
- ❖ For freezing, place the chicken breasts in airtight containers or heavy-duty freezer bags. It will maintain the best quality for about 4 months. Defrost in the refrigerator.
- ❖ Store dressing in your refrigerator for 3 to 4 days. Dress the salad and garnish with fresh avocado. Bon appétit!

## 198) EASY TO COOK RIBS

| Cooking Time: 8 Hours | Servings: 4 |
|---|---|

- ✓ 1 pound baby back ribs
- ✓ 4 tbsp coconut aminos
- ✓ 1/4 cup dry red wine
- ✓ 1/2 tsp cayenne pepper
- ✓ 1 garlic clove, crushed
- ✓ 1 tsp Italian herb mix
- ✓ 1 tbsp butter
- ✓ 1 tsp Serrano pepper, minced
- ✓ 1 Italian pepper, thinly sliced
- ✓ 1 tsp grated lemon zest

- ❖ Butter the sides and bottom of your Crock pot. Place the pork and peppers on the bottom.
- ❖ Add in the remaining ingredients.
- ❖ Slow cook for 9 hours on Low heat setting.
- ❖ Storing
- ❖ Divide the baby back ribs into four portions. Place each portion of the ribs along with the peppers in an airtight container; keep in your refrigerator for 3 to days.
- ❖ For freezing, place the ribs in airtight containers or heavy-duty freezer bags. Freeze up to 4 to months. Defrost in the refrigerator. Reheat in your oven at 250 degrees F until heated through.

## 199) CLASSIC BRIE-STUFFED MEATBALLS

| Cooking Time: 25 Minutes | Servings: 5 |
|---|---|

- ✓ 2 eggs, beaten
- ✓ 1 pound ground pork
- ✓ 1/3 cup double cream
- ✓ 1 tbsp fresh parsley
- ✓ Kosher salt and ground black pepper
- ✓ 1 tsp dried rosemary
- ✓ 10 (1-inch cubes of brie cheese
- ✓ 2 tbsp scallions, minced
- ✓ 2 cloves garlic, minced

- ❖ Mix all ingredients, except for the brie cheese, until everything is well incorporated.
- ❖ Roll the mixture into 10 patties; place a piece of cheese in the center of each patty and roll into a ball.
- ❖ Roast in the preheated oven at 0 degrees F for about 20 minutes.
- ❖ Storing
- ❖ Place the meatballs in airtight containers or Ziploc bags; keep in your refrigerator for up to 3 to 4 days.
- ❖ Freeze the meatballs in airtight containers or heavy-duty freezer bags. Freeze up to 3 to 4 months. To defrost, slowly reheat in a saucepan. Bon appétit!

**Nutrition:** 302 Calories; 13g Fat; 1.9g Carbs; 33.4g Protein; 0.3g Fiber

# Chapter 4. DESSERTS AND SNACKS

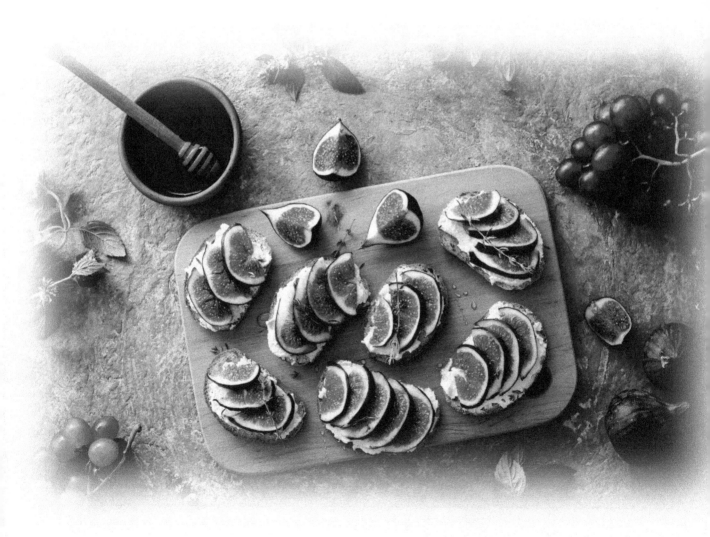

## 200) DELICIOUS SHORTBREAD COOKIES WITH ALMONDS

| | Cooking Time: 25 Minutes | Servings: 16 |
|---|---|---|

**Ingredients:**

- ✓ ½ cup coconut oil
- ✓ 1 tsp vanilla extract
- ✓ 2 egg yolks
- ✓ 1 tbsp brandy
- ✓ 1 cup powdered sugar
- ✓ 1 cup finely ground almonds
- ✓ 3 ½ cups cake flour
- ✓ ½ cup almond butter
- ✓ 1 tbsp water or rose flower water

**Directions:**

- ❖ In a large bowl, combine the coconut oil, powdered sugar, and butter. If the butter is not soft, you want to wait until it softens up. Use an electric mixer to beat the ingredients together at high speed.
- ❖ In a small bowl, add the egg yolks, brandy, water, and vanilla extract. Whisk well.
- ❖ Fold the egg yolk mixture into the large bowl.
- ❖ Add the flour and almonds. Fold and mix with a wooden spoon.
- ❖ Place the mixture into the fridge for at least 1 hour and 30 minutes.
- ❖ Preheat your oven to 325 degrees Fahrenheit.
- ❖ Take the mixture, which now looks like dough, and divide it into 1-inch balls.
- ❖ With a piece of parchment paper on a baking sheet, arrange the cookies and flatten them with a fork or your fingers.
- ❖ Place the cookies in the oven for 13 minutes, but watch them so they don't burn.
- ❖ Transfer the cookies onto a rack to cool for a couple of minutes before enjoying!

**Nutrition:** calories: 250, fats: 14 grams, carbohydrates: 30 grams, protein: 3 grams

## 201) CLASSIC CHOCOLATE FRUIT KEBABS

| | Cooking Time: 30 Minutes | Servings: 6 |
|---|---|---|

**Ingredients:**

- ✓ 24 blueberries
- ✓ 12 strawberries with the green leafy top part removed
- ✓ 12 green or red grapes, seedless
- ✓ 12 pitted cherries
- ✓ 8 ounces chocolate

**Directions:**

- ❖ Line a baking sheet with a piece of parchment paper and place 6, -inch long wooden skewers on top of the paper.
- ❖ Start by threading a piece of fruit onto the skewers. You can create and follow any pattern that you like with the ingredients. An example pattern is 1 strawberry, 1 cherry, blueberries, 2 grapes. Repeat the pattern until all of the fruit is on the skewers.
- ❖ In a saucepan on medium heat, melt the chocolate. Stir continuously until the chocolate has melted completely.
- ❖ Carefully scoop the chocolate into a plastic sandwich bag and twist the bag closed starting right above the chocolate.
- ❖ Snip the corner of the bag with scissors.
- ❖ Drizzle the chocolate onto the kebabs by squeezing it out of the bag.
- ❖ Put the baking pan into the freezer for 20 minutes.
- ❖ Serve and enjoy!

**Nutrition:** calories: 254, fats: 15 grams, carbohydrates: 28 grams, protein: 4 grams
202)

## 203) PEACHES AND BLUE CHEESE CREAM

| **Cooking Time:** 20 Hours 10 Minutes | **Servings:** 4 |
| --- | --- |

**Ingredients:**

- ✓ 4 peaches
- ✓ 1 cinnamon stick
- ✓ 4 ounces sliced blue cheese
- ✓ ⅓ cup orange juice, freshly squeezed is best
- ✓ 3 whole cloves
- ✓ 1 tsp of orange zest, taken from the orange peel
- ✓ ¼ tsp cardamom pods
- ✓ ⅔ cup red wine
- ✓ 2 tbsp honey, raw or your preferred variety
- ✓ 1 vanilla bean
- ✓ 1 tsp allspice berries
- ✓ 4 tbsp dried cherries

**Directions:**

- ❖ Set a saucepan on top of your stove range and add the cinnamon stick, cloves, orange juice, cardamom, vanilla, allspice, red wine, and orange zest. Whisk the ingredients well. Add your peaches to the mixture and poach them for hours or until they become soft.
- ❖ Take a spoon to remove the peaches and boil the rest of the liquid to make the syrup. You want the liquid to reduce itself by at least half.
- ❖ While the liquid is boiling, combine the dried cherries, blue cheese, and honey into a bowl. Once your peaches are cooled, slice them into halves.
- ❖ Top each peach with the blue cheese mixture and then drizzle the liquid onto the top. Serve and enjoy!

**Nutrition:** calories: 211, fats: 24 grams, carbohydrates: 15 grams, protein: 6 grams

## 204) ITALIAN-STYLE BLACKBERRY ICE CREAM

| **Cooking Time:** 15 Minutes | **Servings:** 6 |
| --- | --- |

**Ingredients:**

- ✓ 3 egg yolks
- ✓ 1 container of Greek yogurt
- ✓ 1 pound mashed blackberries
- ✓ ½ tsp vanilla essence
- ✓ 1 tsp arrowroot powder
- ✓ ¼ tsp ground cloves
- ✓ 5 ounces sugar or sweetener substitute
- ✓ 1 pound heavy cream

**Directions:**

- ❖ In a small bowl, add the arrowroot powder and egg yolks. Whisk or beat them with an electronic mixture until they are well combined.
- ❖ Set a saucepan on top of your stove and turn your heat to medium.
- ❖ Add the heavy cream and bring it to a boil.
- ❖ Turn off the heat and add the egg mixture into the cream through folding.
- ❖ Turn the heat back on to medium and pour in the sugar. Cook the mixture for 10 minutes or until it starts to thicken.
- ❖ Remove the mixture from heat and place it in the fridge so it can completely cool. This should take about one hour.
- ❖ Once the mixture is cooled, add in the Greek yogurt, ground cloves, blackberries, and vanilla by folding in the ingredients.
- ❖ Transfer the ice cream into a container and place it in the freezer for at least two hours.
- ❖ Serve and enjoy!

**Nutrition:** calories: 402, fats: 20 grams, carbohydrates: 52 grams, protein: 8 grams

## 205) CLASSIC STUFFED FIGS

| | Cooking Time: 20 Minutes | Servings: 6 |
|---|---|---|

**Ingredients:**

- ✓ 10 halved fresh figs
- ✓ 20 chopped almonds
- ✓ 4 ounces goat cheese, divided
- ✓ 2 tbsp of raw honey

**Directions:**

- ❖ Turn your oven to broiler mode and set it to a high temperature.
- ❖ Place your figs, cut side up, on a baking sheet. If you like to place a piece of parchment paper on top you can do this, but it is not necessary.
- ❖ Sprinkle each fig with half of the goat cheese.
- ❖ Add a tbsp of chopped almonds to each fig.
- ❖ Broil the figs for 3 to 4 minutes.
- ❖ Take them out of the oven and let them cool for 5 to 7 minutes.
- ❖ Sprinkle with the remaining goat cheese and honey.

## 206) CHIA PUDDING AND STRAWBERRIES

| | Cooking Time: 4 Hours 5 Minutes | Servings: 4 |
|---|---|---|

**Ingredients:**

- ✓ 2 cups unsweetened almond milk
- ✓ 1 tbsp vanilla extract
- ✓ 2 tbsp raw honey
- ✓ ¼ cup chia seeds
- ✓ 2 cups fresh and sliced strawberries

**Directions:**

- ❖ In a medium bowl, combine the honey, chia seeds, vanilla, and unsweetened almond milk. Mix well.
- ❖ Set the mixture in the refrigerator for at least 4 hours.
- ❖ When you serve the pudding, top it with strawberries. You can even create a design in a glass serving bowl or dessert dish by adding a little pudding on the bottom, a few strawberries, top the strawberries with some more pudding, and then top the dish with a few strawberries.

## 207) Lovely Strawberry Popsicle

| | Cooking Time: 10 Minutes | Servings: 5 |
|---|---|---|

**Ingredients:**

- ✓ ½ cup almond milk
- ✓ 1 ½ cups fresh strawberries

**Directions:**

- ❖ Using a blender or hand mixer, combine the almond milk and strawberries thoroughly in a bowl.
- ❖ Using popsicle molds, pour the mixture into the molds and place the sticks into the mixture.
- ❖ Set in the freezer for at least 4 hours.
- ❖ Serve and enjoy—especially on a hot day!

## 208) SPECIAL FROZEN BLUEBERRY YOGURT

| | Cooking Time: 30 Minutes | Servings: 6 |
|---|---|---|

**Ingredients:**

- ✓ ⅔ cup honey
- ✓ 2 cups chilled yogurt
- ✓ 1 pint fresh blueberries
- ✓ 1 juiced and zested lime or lemon. You can even substitute an orange if your tastes prefer.

**Directions:**

- ❖ With a saucepan on your burner set to medium heat, add the honey, juiced fruit, zest, and blueberries.
- ❖ Stir the mixture continuously as it begins to simmer for 15 minutes.
- ❖ When the liquid is nearly gone, pour the contents into a bowl and place in the fridge for several minutes. You will want to stir the ingredients and check to see if they are chilled.
- ❖ Once the fruit is chilled, combine with the yogurt.
- ❖ Mix until the ingredients are well incorporated and enjoy.

**Nutrition:** calories: 233, fats: 3 grams, carbohydrates: 52 grams, protein: 3.5 grams

# Chapter 5. *THE BEST RECIPES*

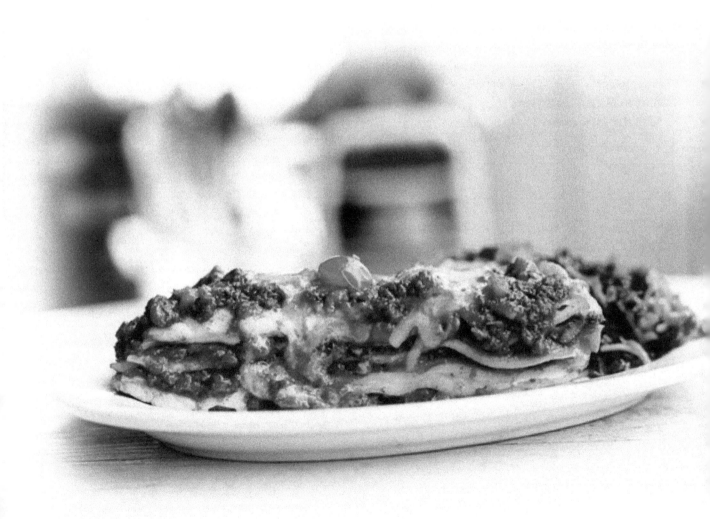

## 209) ITALIAN BAKED ZUCCHINI WITH THYME AND PARMESAN

| Preparation Time: 10 minutes | Cooking Time: 20 minutes | Servings: 4 |
|---|---|---|

**Ingredients:**

- ✓ Four sliced zucchinis
- ✓ 1/2 tsp dried thyme
- ✓ 1/2 cup shredded Parmesan cheese
- ✓ 1/2 tsp dried oregano
- ✓ 2 tbsp olive oil
- ✓ 1/4 tsp garlic powder
- ✓ Kosher salt to taste
- ✓ 1/2 tsp dried basil
- ✓ Black pepper to taste
- ✓ 2 tbsp chopped parsley

**Directions:**

- ❖ Mix all the ingredients in a large bowl except zucchini.
- ❖ Make a layer of zucchini over a baking sheet sprayed with oil.
- ❖ Transfer the cheese mixture over zucchini and pour olive oil over them.
- ❖ Bake in a preheated oven at 350 degrees for 15 minutes, followed by broiling for three minutes.
- ❖ Serve and enjoy it.

## 210) ITALIAN BABA GANOUSH

| Preparation Time: 10 minutes | Cooking Time: 40 minutes | Servings: 4 |
|---|---|---|

**Ingredients:**

- ✓ One eggplant
- ✓ 1 tbsp Greek yogurt
- ✓ olive oil
- ✓ 1.5 tbsp tahini paste
- ✓ 1 tbsp lime juice
- ✓ One garlic clove
- ✓ Salt to taste
- ✓ 1 tsp cayenne pepper
- ✓ Pepper to taste
- ✓ ½ tsp sumac for garnishing
- ✓ Parsley leaves for garnishing
- ✓ Toasted pine nuts for garnishing

**Directions:**

- ❖ Make slits in eggplant's skin.
- ❖ Place eggplant skin side upwards in a baking tray.
- ❖ Spray olive oil over eggplant.
- ❖ Bake in a preheated oven at 425 degrees for 40 minutes.
- ❖ Scoop the inner flesh of eggplant out and shift in a food processor. Add garlic, cayenne, yogurt, lime juice, salt, tahini, sumac, pepper, and blend. The baba ganoush is ready.
- ❖ You can refrigerator for better results for 60 minutes and sprinkle oil, sumac, parsley, and nuts and serve.

## 211) SICILIAN SALMON FISH STICKS

| Preparation Time: 10 minutes | Cooking Time: 18 minutes | Servings: 4 |
|---|---|---|

**Ingredients:**

- ✓ Fish Sticks
- ✓ 2 lb salmon fillet
- ✓ 1/4 tsp salt
- ✓ 1/4 tsp black pepper
- ✓ First coating
- ✓ 1/2 tsp garlic powder
- ✓ 1/2 tsp dried thyme
- ✓ 1 cup almond meal
- ✓ 1/2 tsp sea salt
- ✓ 1/4 tsp black pepper
- ✓ Second coating
- ✓ 1/2 tsp salt
- ✓ 2/3 cup chickpea flour
- ✓ Third coating
- ✓ Two eggs
- ✓ Dipping Sauce
- ✓ 1/4 tsp salt
- ✓ 1/4 cup Greek yogurt
- ✓ 1 tsp lemon juice
- ✓ 1 tbsp Dijon mustard
- ✓ 1/2 tsp dill
- ✓ 1/8 tsp garlic powder

**Directions:**

- ❖ Whisk all the ingredients for the dipping sauce list in a bowl and set aside. The dipping sauce is ready.
- ❖ Mix garlic, thyme, and almond meal in a bowl. The first coating is ready.
- ❖ Add chickpea flour in another bowl. The second coating is ready.
- ❖ Beat the eggs in another bowl. Set aside.
- ❖ Sprinkle pepper and salt over sliced fish with removed skin.
- ❖ First, coat the fish with chickpea flour, followed by coating with egg and almond meal coating.
- ❖ Aline coated fish pieces in a baking sheet covered with parchment paper.
- ❖ Bake in a preheated oven at 400 degrees for 18 minutes.
- ❖ Serve baked fish with dipping sauce and serve.

**Nutrition:** Calories: 92 kcal Fat: 5.7 g Protein: 14.4 g Carbs: 4.5 g Fiber: 1.3 g

| 212) | AFRICAN BAKED FALAFEL | |
|---|---|---|
| **Preparation Time:** 10 minutes | **Cooking Time:** 24 minutes | **Servings: 15 patties** |

**Ingredients:**

- ✓ 15 oz chickpeas
- ✓ Three cloves garlic
- ✓ 1/4 cup chopped onion
- ✓ 1/2 cup parsley
- ✓ 2 tsp lemon juice
- ✓ 1/2 tsp baking soda
- ✓ 1 tbsp olive oil
- ✓ 1 tsp ground cumin
- ✓ 3/4 tsp salt
- ✓ 1 tsp coriander
- ✓ One pinch of cayenne
- ✓ 3 tbsp oat flour

**Directions:**

- ❖ Blend all the ingredients except oat flour and baking soda in a food processor to get roughly a blended mixture.
- ❖ Transfer the mixture to a bowl and add oat flour and baking soda. Using hands, mix the dough well.
- ❖ Make patties out of the falafel mixture and set aside for 15 minutes.
- ❖ Bake the falafel patties in a preheated oven at 375 degrees for 12 minutes and serve.

**Nutrition:** Calories: 143 kcal Fat: 5 g Protein: 6 g Carbs: 24 g Fiber: 6 g

| 213) | GREEK CHIA YOGURT PUDDING | |
|---|---|---|
| **Preparation Time:** 10 minutes | **Cooking Time:** 0 minute | **Servings: 4** |

**Ingredients:**

- ✓ 3/4 cup milk
- ✓ 11 oz f Vanilla Yogurt
- ✓ 2 tbsp pure maple syrup
- ✓ 1 tsp vanilla extract
- ✓ 1/8 tsp salt
- ✓ 1/4 cup chia seeds
- ✓ Sliced almonds for garnishing

**Directions:**

- ❖ Whisk all the ingredients in a large bowl. Set aside for 24 hours in the refrigerator.
- ❖ Mix the mixture gently after 24 hours and serve after garnishing.

**Nutrition:** Calories: 179 kcal Fat: 5.6 g Protein: 10.1 g Carbs: 22.3 g Fiber: 6 g

| 214) | EASY ITALIAN-STYLE FARFALLE | |
|---|---|---|
| **Preparation Time:** 10 minutes | **Cooking Time:** 15 minutes | **Servings: 7** |

**Ingredients:**

- ✓ 12 oz farfalle pasta
- ✓ ½ cup olive oil
- ✓ ¼ cup chopped basil leaves
- ✓ 1 lb crumbled chorizo sausage
- ✓ ½ cup pine nuts
- ✓ ½ cup shredded parmesan cheese
- ✓ Two chopped garlic cloves
- ✓ 1 cup diced tomato
- ✓ ¼ cup red wine vinegar

**Directions:**

- ❖ In a saucepan, boil water with added salt.
- ❖ Add pasta and cook until pasta is done.
- ❖ In a pan, cook chorizo over medium flame. Stir in nuts and cook for five minutes.
- ❖ Mix garlic and cook for a minute before removing the pan from the flame.
- ❖ Transfer cooked pasta, vinegar, cheese, cooked chorizo mixture, olive oil, tomatoes, and basil. Mix well to coat everything and serve.

**Nutrition:** Calories: 692 kcal Fat: 48 g Protein: 26.9 g Carbs: 39.7 g Fiber: 15 g

## 215)  SPECIAL POTATO WEDGES

| Preparation Time: 5 minutes | Cooking Time: 30 minutes | Servings: 4 |
|---|---|---|

| Ingredients: | | Directions: |
|---|---|---|
| ✓ Two wedges cut potatoes<br>✓ ½ tsp salt<br>✓ ½ tsp paprika | ✓ 1.5 tbsp olive oil<br>✓ ½ tsp chili powder<br>✓ 1/8 black pepper | ❖ Combine all the ingredients in a bowl.<br>❖ Transfer the mixture to an air fryer basket and cook in a preheated air fryer at 400 degrees for eight minutes from both sides.<br>❖ Serve and enjoy it. |

## 216)  ORIGINAL GREEK-STYLE POTATOES

| Preparation Time: 20 minutes | Cooking Time: 120 minutes | Servings: 4 |
|---|---|---|

| Ingredients: | | Directions: |
|---|---|---|
| ✓ 1/3 cup olive oil<br>✓ Two chopped garlic cloves<br>✓ 1.5 cups water<br>✓ Black pepper to taste | ✓ ¼ cup lemon juice<br>✓ 1 tsp rosemary<br>✓ 1 tsp thyme<br>✓ Two chicken bouillon cubes<br>✓ Six chopped potatoes | ❖ Mix all the ingredients in a large bowl and pour over the potatoes placed in the baking tray.<br>❖ Bake in a preheated oven at 350 degrees for 90 minutes.<br>❖ Serve and enjoy it. |

## 217)  ORGINIAL ITALIAN-STYLE CHICKEN WRAP

| Preparation Time: 10 minutes | Cooking Time: 20 minutes | Servings: 4 |
|---|---|---|

| Ingredients: | | Directions: |
|---|---|---|
| ✓ 2 tbsp butter<br>✓ 1/2 cup mayonnaise<br>✓ 1/2 lb boneless chicken breasts<br>✓ 1/4 cup shredded Parmesan cheese<br>✓ 2 cups shredded romaine lettuce | ✓ Four flour tortillas<br>✓ Two sliced Roma tomatoes<br>✓ 1/2 cup crushed croutons<br>✓ 16 basil leaves | ❖ Cook chicken over medium flame in melted butter for 20 minutes.<br>❖ Slice the chicken into strips.<br>❖ Whisk cheese and mayonnaise and pour over the tortilla.<br>❖ Place lettuce followed by chicken, basil, tomato, and croutons on tortilla and wrap.<br>❖ Serve and enjoy it. |

## 218)  Lovely Avocado Caprese wrap

| Preparation Time: 20 minutes | Cooking Time: 0 minute | Servings: 3 |
|---|---|---|

| Ingredients: | | Directions: |
|---|---|---|
| ✓ Two tortillas<br>✓ Balsamic vinegar as needed<br>✓ One ball mozzarella cheese grated<br>✓ 1/2 cup arugula leaves<br>✓ One sliced tomato | ✓ 2 tbsp basil leaves<br>✓ Kosher salt to taste<br>✓ One sliced avocado<br>✓ Olive oil as required<br>✓ Black pepper to taste | ❖ Place tomato slices and cheese, followed by avocado and basil. Over one side of the tortilla.<br>❖ Pour olive oil and vinegar. Drizzle pepper and salt.<br>❖ Wrap the tortilla and serve. |

## 219) DELICIOUS CHICKEN SALAD WITH AVOCADO AND GREEK YOGURT

| Preparation Time: 10 minutes | Cooking Time: 0 minute | Servings: 4 |
| --- | --- | --- |

**Ingredients:**

- ✓ 1 cup plain yogurt
- ✓ 1 tbsp lemon juice
- ✓ One mashed avocado
- ✓ 1/3 cup dried cranberries
- ✓ Kosher salt to taste
- ✓ 2 cups shredded chicken
- ✓ Black pepper to taste
- ✓ 3/4 cup chopped celery
- ✓ 1/3 cup chopped pecans
- ✓ 1/2 cup chopped red grapes
- ✓ 1/3 cup chopped red onion
- ✓ 2 tbsp chopped tarragon

**Directions:**

- ❖ Whisk all the ingredients in a large mixing bowl.
- ❖ Serve as a salad and enjoy it.

## 220) EASY CHICKEN SHAWARMA PITAS

| Preparation Time: 10 minutes | Cooking Time: 30 minutes | Servings: 6 |
| --- | --- | --- |

- ✓ ¾ tbsp cumin
- ✓ ¾ tbsp coriander
- ✓ ¾ tbsp turmeric powder
- ✓ One sliced onion
- ✓ ¾ tbsp garlic powder
- ✓ ½ tsp cloves
- ✓ ¾ tbsp paprika
- ✓ 1 tbsp lemon juice
- ✓ ½ tsp cayenne pepper
- ✓ Eight boneless chicken
- ✓ Salt to taste
- ✓ 1/3 cup olive oil
- ✓ Pita bread
- ✓ Tahini sauce

**Directions:**

- ❖ In a bowl, add sliced chicken pieces, onions, cumin, garlic, cloves, olive oil, turmeric, paprika, lemon juice, salt, and coriander. Toss well to coat chicken evenly. Set aside for three hours in the refrigerator.
- ❖ Transfer the chicken pieces along with the marinade in a baking tray sprayed with oil.
- ❖ Bake in a preheated oven at 425 degrees for 30 minutes.
- ❖ Spread tahini sauce in pita bread and add baked chicken pieces. You can also add your favorite salad.
- ❖ Serve and enjoy it.

## 221) SIMPLE RED LENTIL SOUP

| Preparation Time: 10 minutes | Cooking Time: 45 minutes | Servings: 4 |
| --- | --- | --- |

- ✓ Four minced garlic cloves
- ✓ ¼ cup olive oil
- ✓ 1 tsp curry powder
- ✓ Two chopped carrots
- ✓ 2 tsp ground cumin
- ✓ One chopped onion
- ✓ ½ tsp dried thyme
- ✓ 1 cup brown lentils
- ✓ 28 oz diced tomatoes
- ✓ 4 cups vegetable broth
- ✓ 1 tsp salt
- ✓ 2 cups of water
- ✓ One pinch of red pepper flakes
- ✓ 1 cup chopped kale
- ✓ Black pepper to taste
- ✓ 1.5 tbsp lemon juice

**Directions:**

- ❖ Cook carrots and onions in ¼ cup of heated olive oil in a Dutch oven over medium flame for five minutes.
- ❖ Stir in thyme, cumin, garlic, and curry powder,
- ❖ Cook for half a minute.
- ❖ Add tomatoes and cook for another five minutes.
- ❖ Add pepper flakes, broth, salt, lentils, black pepper, and water in a Dutch oven.
- ❖ Let it boil. Cover the oven and lower the flame and let it simmer for 30 minutes.
- ❖ Blend a portion of soup of about two cups in a food processor and transfer it into the pot again.
- ❖ Mix chopped greens and cook for another five minutes.
- ❖ Remove from the flame and mix lemon juice and serve.

**Nutrition:** Calories: 366 kcal Fat: 15.5 g Protein: 14.5 g Carbs: 47.8 g Fiber: 10.8 g

## 222) EASY SALMON SOUP

| Preparation Time: 10 minutes | Cooking Time: 12 minutes | Servings: 4 |
|---|---|---|

**Ingredients:**

- Olive oil
- ½ chopped green bell pepper
- Four chopped green onions
- Four minced garlic cloves
- 5 cups chicken broth
- 1 oz chopped dill
- 1 lb sliced gold potatoes
- 1 tsp dry oregano
- One sliced carrot
- ¾ tsp coriander
- Kosher salt to taste
- ½ tsp cumin
- Black pepper to taste
- Zest of one lemon
- 1 lb sliced salmon fillet
- 1 tbsp lemon juice

**Directions:**

- ❖ Cook onions, garlic, and bell pepper in heated olive oil in a pot over medium flame for four minutes.
- ❖ Stir in the dill and cook for half a minute.
- ❖ Pour broth into the pot. Add carrot, potatoes, salt, spices, and pepper.
- ❖ Let it boil. Reduce the flame and let it simmer for six minutes.
- ❖ Add salmon and cook for five more minutes.
- ❖ Add lemon juice and zest and cook for one minute.
- ❖ Serve the soup and enjoy it.

## 223) RICH FALAFEL SANDWICHES

| Preparation Time: 20 minutes | Cooking Time: 10 minutes | Servings: 4 sandwiches |
|---|---|---|

**Ingredients:**

- 4 Pita Breads
- 1 cup arugula
- 1 tbsp lemon
- 1/2 cup tahini sauce
- 12 falafels
- One sliced red onion
- 1/2 cup tabbouleh salad
- Three sprigs mint

**Directions:**

- ❖ Spread tahini sauce followed by the addition of arugula and crushed falafels over pita bread.
- ❖ Add tabbouleh salad, mint, and onions over pita and drizzle lemon juice.
- ❖ Wrap the pita bread and serve.

## 224) EASY ROASTED TOMATO AND BASIL SOUP

| Preparation Time: 10 minutes | Cooking Time: 50 minutes | Servings: 6 |
|---|---|---|

**Ingredients:**

- 3 lb halved Roma tomatoes
- Olive oil
- Two chopped carrots
- Salt to taste
- Two chopped yellow onions
- Black pepper to taste
- Five minced garlic cloves
- 2 oz basil leaves
- 1 cup crushed tomatoes
- Three thyme sprigs
- 1 tsp dry oregano
- 2 tsp thyme leaves
- ½ tsp paprika
- 2.5 cups water
- ½ tsp cumin
- 1 tbsp lime juice

**Directions:**

- ❖ Mix salt, olive oil, carrot, black pepper, and tomatoes in a bowl.
- ❖ Transfer carrot mixture to a baking tray and bake in a preheated oven at 450 degrees for 30 minutes.
- ❖ Blend baked tomato mixture in a blender. You can use a little water if needed during blending.
- ❖ Sauté onions in heated olive oil over medium flame in a pot for three minutes.
- ❖ Mix garlic and cook for one more minute.
- ❖ Transfer the blended tomato mixture to the pot, followed by the addition of crushed tomatoes, water, spices, thyme, salt, basil, and pepper.
- ❖ Let it boil. Reduce the flame and simmer for 20 minutes.
- ❖ Drizzle lemon juice and serve.

## 225) GREEK-STYLE BLACK-EYED PEAS STEW

| Preparation Time: 5 minutes | Cooking Time: 55 minutes | Servings: 6 |
|---|---|---|

**Ingredients:**

- ✓ Olive oil
- ✓ Four chopped garlic cloves
- ✓ 30 oz black-eyed peas
- ✓ One chopped yellow onion
- ✓ One chopped green bell pepper
- ✓ 15 oz diced tomato
- ✓ Three chopped carrots
- ✓ 1.5 tsp cumin
- ✓ One dry bay leaf
- ✓ 1 tsp dry oregano
- ✓ Kosher salt to taste
- ✓ ½ tsp red pepper flakes
- ✓ ½ tsp paprika
- ✓ Black pepper to taste
- ✓ 1 cup chopped parsley
- ✓ 1 tbsp of lime juice
- ✓ 2 cups of water

**Directions:**

- ❖ Cook garlic and onions in a heated oven in a Dutch oven over medium flame for five minutes with constant stirring.
- ❖ Stir in tomatoes, pepper, water, spices, bay leaf, and salt.
- ❖ Let it boil.
- ❖ Mix black-eyed beans and cook for five more minutes.
- ❖ Cover the oven and reduce the flame. Simmer for 30 minutes.
- ❖ Squeeze lemon juice and mix.
- ❖ Serve and enjoy.

## 226) GREEK CHICKEN GYROS WITH TZATZIKI SAUCE

| Preparation Time: 10 minutes | Cooking Time: 8 minutes | Servings: 4 |
|---|---|---|

**Ingredients:**

- ✓ Greek Chicken
- ✓ 1 tbsp lemon juice
- ✓ 1/2 cup plain yogurt
- ✓ 1.25 tsp Italian-spiced salt
- ✓ 2 tbsp extra-virgin olive oil
- ✓ 1 cup Tzatziki sauce
- ✓ Four slices of pita bread
- ✓ Four chopped tomatoes
- ✓ 1/4 sliced red onion
- ✓ Tzatziki Sauce
- ✓ ½ halved cucumber
- ✓ ¾ cup Greek yogurt
- ✓ Two minced garlic cloves
- ✓ 1 tbsp red wine vinegar
- ✓ 1 tbsp chopped dill
- ✓ One pinch of kosher salt
- ✓ One pinch of black pepper

**Directions:**

- ❖ Marinate the chicken by mixing it with lemon juice, salt, and yogurt. Set aside for one hour.
- ❖ Heat olive oil in a skillet over medium flame.
- ❖ Add chicken without marinade and cook for five minutes from both sides. Transfer the cooked brown chicken to the plate.
- ❖ Mix all the ingredients of Tzatziki sauce in a bowl and set aside. The Tzatziki sauce is ready.
- ❖ Toast pita bread and place Tzatziki sauce, tomatoes, onions, and chicken pieces over pita bread. Wrap and serve.

**Nutrition:** Calories: 411 kcal Fat: 21 g Protein: 44 g Carbs: 10 g Fiber: 1 g

## 227)  GREEK-STYLE CHICKEN MARINADE

| Preparation Time:  5 minutes | Cooking Time:  15 minutes | Servings: 4 |
|---|---|---|

**Ingredients:**

- ✓ 1 lb boneless chicken breasts
- ✓ ¼ cup olive oil
- ✓ ½ tsp black pepper
- ✓ 1/3 cup Greek yogurt
- ✓ Four lemons
- ✓ 2 tbsp dried oregano
- ✓ Five minced garlic cloves
- ✓ 1 tsp kosher salt

**Directions:**

- ❖ Mix all the ingredients in a bowl and set aside for three hours.
- ❖ Preheat the grill and grill chicken and lemon slices for 20 minutes from both sides.
- ❖ Slice the grilled chicken and serve.

**Nutrition:** Calories: 304 kcal Fat: 19 g Protein: 25 g Carbs: 14 g Fiber: 4 g

## 228)  ITALIAN STYLE CHICKEN QUINOA BOWL WITH BROCCOLI AND TOMATO

| Preparation Time:  10 minutes | Cooking Time:  30 minutes | Servings: 3 |
|---|---|---|

**Ingredients:**

- ✓ Chicken
- ✓ 6 oz boneless chicken breast
- ✓ 1 cup Easy Roasted Feta and Broccoli
- ✓ 1/2 cup olive oil
- ✓ 1/2 tsp kosher salt
- ✓ Zest of one lemon
- ✓ 2 tsp dried oregano
- ✓ 1.5 tbsp lemon juice
- ✓ 1/4 tsp black pepper
- ✓ Two minced garlic cloves
- ✓ 1/2 cup Easy Roasted Tomatoes
- ✓ Quinoa
- ✓ 1 tsp kosher salt
- ✓ 1 cup dried quinoa
- ✓ Feta cheese to taste

**Directions:**

- ❖ Mix lemon juice, oregano, salt, olive oil, garlic, lemon zest, and pepper in a bowl.
- ❖ Add chicken and toss well. Set aside for one hour.
- ❖ Cook chicken in heat olive oil over medium flame for 15 minutes.
- ❖ Lower the flame and stir in tomatoes and broccoli and cook. Set aside.
- ❖ Add water and salt to a pot and bring it to a boil.
- ❖ Add quinoa and cook for ten minutes.
- ❖ Drain the quinoa and set aside.
- ❖ Add quinoa in a bowl, followed by the addition of chicken and veggies. Sprinkle salt, cheese, oil, and pepper.
- ❖ Serve and enjoy it.

**Nutrition:** Calories: 481 kcal Fat: 23 g Protein: 24 g Carbs: 45 g Fiber: 7 g

## 229)  EASY CHICKEN PICCATA

| Preparation Time:  10 minutes | Cooking Time:  10 minutes | Servings: 4 |
|---|---|---|

**Ingredients:**

- ✓ 1.5 lb boneless chicken breasts
- ✓ One lemon
- ✓ 2 tbsp canola oil
- ✓ 1 tsp kosher salt
- ✓ 1 cup chicken broth
- ✓ 1 tsp black pepper
- ✓ 2 tbsp capers
- ✓ 3 tbsp butter
- ✓ 1/3 cup all-purpose flour

**Directions:**

- ❖ Mix salt, flour, and pepper in a bowl. Coat chicken with the flour mixture. Set aside.
- ❖ Cook chicken pieces in heated butter and canola oil over medium flame for five minutes from both sides. Shift cooked pieces onto the plate.
- ❖ Lower the flame and pour broth and add sliced lemon, butter (1 tbsp), lemon juice, capers, and cook for five minutes.
- ❖ Pour the sauce over chicken pieces and serve with cauliflower or noodles.

**Nutrition:** Calories: 381 kcal Fat: 20 g Protein: 37 g Carbs: 11 g Fiber: 1 g

## 230) ITALIAN CHOPPED GRILLED VEGETABLE WITH FARRO

| Preparation Time: 5 minutes | Cooking Time: 50 minutes | Servings: 2 |
|---|---|---|

**Ingredients:**

- ✓ 1 cup dried farro
- ✓ 1 Portobello mushroom
- ✓ 3 cups vegetable broth
- ✓ One sliced red bell pepper
- ✓ 1/2 sliced red onion
- ✓ 8 oz asparagus
- ✓ One sliced zucchini
- ✓ Olive oil as required
- ✓ 1/4 cup halved Kalamata olives
- ✓ One sliced yellow squash
- ✓ Kosher salt to taste
- ✓ 1-pint Greek yogurt
- ✓ Black pepper to taste
- ✓ 2 tbsp minced cucumber
- ✓ One chopped garlic clove
- ✓ 1 tbsp lemon juice
- ✓ 1 tsp chopped dill
- ✓ 1 tsp chopped mint
- ✓ Red bell pepper hummus
- ✓ 1/8 cup feta cheese

**Directions:**

- ❖ In a large pot, add broth and farro. Let it boil over a high flame.
- ❖ Lower the flame to medium and cook for half an hour with occasional stirring.
- ❖ Mix veggies with salt, olive oil, and pepper.
- ❖ Grill the veggies in a preheated grill until marks appear on them. Keep them aside.
- ❖ Whisk cucumber, salt, mint, dill, yogurt, lemon juice, and garlic in a bowl.
- ❖ Make the layers of farro, grilled veggies, hummus, olives, and cheese.
- ❖ Pour yogurt sauce and sprinkle mint and serve.

**Nutrition:** Calories: 140 kcal Fat: 6 g Protein: 4 g Carbs: 20 g Fiber: 5 g

## 231) QUICK PORK ESCALOPES IN 30 MINUTES WITH LEMONS AND CAPERS

| Preparation Time: 10 minutes | Cooking Time: 20 minutes | Servings: 4 |
|---|---|---|

**Ingredients:**

- ✓ Four boneless pork chops
- ✓ 1/4 cup all-purpose flour
- ✓ Eight sage leaves
- ✓ kosher salt to taste
- ✓ 2 tbsp chopped parsley
- ✓ 4 tbsp butter
- ✓ Black pepper to taste
- ✓ 1 tbsp vegetable oil
- ✓ 1/4 cup capers
- ✓ 1/2 cup white wine
- ✓ 1 cup chicken stock
- ✓ One sliced lemon
- ✓ 4 tbsp lemon juice

**Directions:**

- ❖ One each pork chops, place two sage leaves on both sides. Set aside.
- ❖ In a bowl, whisk salt, flour, and pepper.
- ❖ Coat pork chops with flour. Keep the sage leaves in place.
- ❖ Melt butter in a skillet over medium flame.
- ❖ Cook pork chops for five minutes from both sides.
- ❖ Clean the skillet and melt butter in it.
- ❖ Pour wine and add capers in skillet. Cook to concentrate the wine.
- ❖ Pour stock, lemon slices, and lemon juice. Let it boil for five more minutes.
- ❖ Place pork in sauce and cook for two minutes.
- ❖ Sprinkle parsley and serve.

**Nutrition:** Calories: 415 kcal Fat: 7 g Protein: 31 g Carbs: 14 g Fiber: 8 g

## 232) GREEK-STYLE CHICKEN KEBABS

| Preparation Time: 40 minutes | Cooking Time: 15 minutes | Servings: 6 |
|---|---|---|

**Ingredients:**

- ✓ 1 lb boneless chicken breasts
- ✓ 1/4 cup olive oil
- ✓ One sliced red bell pepper
- ✓ 1/3 cup Greek yogurt
- ✓ 10 tbsp lemons juice
- ✓ Four chopped garlic cloves
- ✓ Zest of one lemon
- ✓ 2 tbsp dried oregano
- ✓ 1/2 tsp black pepper
- ✓ One sliced zucchini
- ✓ 1 tsp kosher salt
- ✓ One sliced red onion

**Directions:**

- ❖ Whisk all the ingredients except chicken in a bowl. Add chicken and toss to coat chicken evenly. Set aside four hours for better results.
- ❖ Thread chicken, zucchini, onion, and bell pepper on the skewers.
- ❖ Grill the chicken, skewers on a preheated grill for 15 minutes, occasionally turning and basting with marinade.

**Nutrition:** Calories: 224 kcal Fat: 13 g Protein: 18 g Carbs: 13 g Fiber: 4 g

## 233) EASY PASTA WITH SHRIMP AND ROASTED RED PEPPERS AND ARTICHOKES

| Preparation Time: 10 minutes | Cooking Time: 25 minutes | Servings: 8 |
|---|---|---|

**Ingredients:**

- ✓ 12 oz farfalle pasta
- ✓ 1/4 cup butter
- ✓ 1.5 lb shrimp
- ✓ Three chopped garlic cloves
- ✓ 1 cup sliced artichoke hearts
- ✓ 12 oz roasted and chopped red bell peppers
- ✓ 1/2 cup dry white wine
- ✓ 1/4 cup basil
- ✓ 1/2 cup whipping cream
- ✓ 3 tbsp drained capers
- ✓ 1 tsp grated lemon peel
- ✓ 3/4 cup feta cheese
- ✓ 2 tbsp lemon juice
- ✓ 2 oz toasted pine nuts

**Directions:**

- ❖ Boil water in a pot and cook pasta in it.
- ❖ Drain pasta and set aside.
- ❖ Melt butter in a skillet over medium flame. Sauté garlic and cook for one minute.
- ❖ Stir in shrimps and cook for about two minutes.
- ❖ Mix artichokes, capers, bell pepper, and wine. Let it boil.
- ❖ Lower the flame and let it simmer for two minutes with occasional stirring.
- ❖ Add whipping cream, lemon juice, and lemon zest.
- ❖ Let it boil for five minutes.
- ❖ Transfer the cooked shrimps over pasta and mix well.
- ❖ Spread cheese, basil, and nuts and serve.

**Nutrition:** Calories: 627 kcal Fat: 24 g Protein: 38 g Carbs: 58 g Fiber: 3 g

## 234)     CHICKEN CAPRESE QUICK IN 30 MINUTES

| **Preparation Time:** 10 minutes | **Cooking Time:** 20 minutes | **Servings: 4** |
|---|---|---|

**Ingredients:**

- ✓ Two boneless chicken breasts
- ✓ Black pepper to taste
- ✓ 1 tbsp butter
- ✓ 1 tbsp extra virgin olive oil
- ✓ 6 oz Pesto
- ✓ Eight chopped tomatoes
- ✓ Six grated mozzarella cheese
- ✓ Balsamic glaze as needed
- ✓ Kosher salt to taste
- ✓ Basil as required

**Directions:**

- ❖ Mix salt, sliced chicken, and pepper in a bowl. Set aside for ten minutes.
- ❖ Melt butter in a skillet over medium flame.
- ❖ Cook chicken pieces in melted butter for five minutes from both sides.
- ❖ Remove from the flame. Sprinkle pesto and place mozzarella cheese and tomatoes over chicken pieces.
- ❖ Bake in a preheated oven at 400 degrees for 12 minutes.
- ❖ Garnish with balsamic glaze and serve.

**Nutrition:** Calories: 232 kcal Fat: 15 g Protein: 18 g Carbs: 5 g Fiber: 1 g

## 235)     SPECIAL GRILLED LEMON CHICKEN SKEWERS

| **Preparation Time:** 10 minutes | **Cooking Time:** 10 minutes | **Servings: 6** |
|---|---|---|

**Ingredients:**

- ✓ Two boneless chicken breasts
- ✓ Seven green onions
- ✓ Four minced garlic cloves
- ✓ Three lemons
- ✓ 1 tbsp dried oregano
- ✓ 1 tsp kosher salt
- ✓ 1/4 cup olive oil
- ✓ 1/2 tsp black pepper

**Directions:**

- ❖ Whisk salt, lemon juice, olive oil, garlic, lemon zest, black pepper, oregano, and sliced chicken pieces in a bowl. Set aside for four hours.
- ❖ Thread chicken, onions, and lemon slices onto the skewer.
- ❖ Grill chicken skewers for 15 minutes on preheated grill over medium flames with often turning.
- ❖ Serve when chicken is fully cooked.

## 236)     TASTY JUICY SALMON BURGERS

| **Preparation Time:** 10 minutes | **Cooking Time:** 4 minutes | **Servings: 4** |
|---|---|---|

- ✓ 1.5 lb sliced salmon fillet
- ✓ 3 tbsp minced green onions
- ✓ 1 tsp coriander
- ✓ 2 tsp Dijon mustard
- ✓ 1/3 cup bread crumbs
- ✓ 1 tsp sumac
- ✓ 1 cup chopped parsley
- ✓ ½ tsp sweet paprika
- ✓ Kosher Salt to taste
- ✓ ¼ cup olive oil
- ✓ ½ tsp black pepper
- ✓ One lemon
- ✓ Toppings
- ✓ One sliced red onion
- ✓ Tzatziki Sauce
- ✓ One sliced tomato
- ✓ 6 oz baby arugula

**Directions:**

- ❖ Blend mustard and salmon in a blender.
- ❖ Shift the mixture in a container. Add all the spices, parsley, salt, and onions. Mix well and set aside for 30 minutes.
- ❖ Make patties out of salmon mixture and place in a tray.
- ❖ Coat all the patties with bread crumbs from both sides.
- ❖ Fry the patties in heated olive oil over medium flame for five minutes each from both sides.
- ❖ Drizzle lemon juice over the cooked patties.
- ❖ Spread Tzatziki sauce over the bun, followed by the layer of salmon, arugula, onions, and tomatoes. The salmon burgers are ready. Serve and enjoy it.

## 237) SPECIAL BRAISED EGGPLANT AND CHICKPEAS

| Preparation Time: 20 minutes | Cooking Time: 55 minutes | Servings: 6 |
|---|---|---|

**Ingredients:**

- ✓ 1.5 lb chopped eggplant
- ✓ Olive Oil
- ✓ Kosher salt
- ✓ One chopped yellow onion
- ✓ One chopped carrot
- ✓ One diced green bell pepper
- ✓ Six minced garlic cloves
- ✓ 1.5 tsp sweet paprika
- ✓ Two dry bay leaves
- ✓ 1 tsp organic coriander
- ✓ ¾ tsp cinnamon
- ✓ 1 tsp dry oregano
- ✓ ½ tsp organic turmeric
- ✓ 28 oz chopped tomato
- ✓ ½ tsp black pepper
- ✓ 30 oz chickpeas
- ✓ Handful parsley and mint for garnishing

**Directions:**

- ❖ Sauté onions, carrots, and bell peppers in heated olive oil over medium flame for four minutes with constant stirring.
- ❖ Stir in salt, bay leaf, garlic, and spices and cook for one minute.
- ❖ Mix eggplant, chickpeas, tomato, and chickpea liquid.
- ❖ Let it boil for ten minutes.
- ❖ Remove the pan from flame and cover.
- ❖ Now, bake in a preheated oven at 400 degrees for 45 minutes.
- ❖ Sprinkle herbs and serve with any sauce.

**Nutrition:** Calories: 240 kcal Fat: 5.1 g Protein: 10.6 g Carbs: 42 g Fiber: 15 g

## 238) ITALIAN STYLE TUNA SALAD SANDWICHES

| Preparation Time: 5 minutes | Cooking Time: 0 minute | Servings: 4 |
|---|---|---|

**Ingredients:**

- ✓ 4 tsp red wine vinegar
- ✓ 4 tsp olive oil
- ✓ Eight bread slices
- ✓ ¼ cup chopped red onion
- ✓ 1/3 cup chopped sun-dried tomatoes
- ✓ ¼ tsp black pepper
- ✓ ¼ cup sliced olives
- ✓ 3 tbsp mayonnaise
- ✓ 2 tsp capers
- ✓ Four lettuce leaves
- ✓ 12 oz tuna

**Directions:**

- ❖ Mix wine and olive oil.
- ❖ Brush bread from both sides with oil mixture.
- ❖ Mix all the ingredients except lettuce and bread slices in a bowl.
- ❖ Place lettuce on each bread slices brushed with oil. Spread tuna mixture and cover with second bread piece and serve.

**Nutrition:** Calories: 293 kcal Fat: 10 g Protein: 21.2 g Carbs: 31.3 g Fiber: 4.6 g

## 239) MOROCCAN-STYLE VEGETABLE TAGINE

| Preparation Time: 15 minutes | Cooking Time: 40 minutes | Servings: 5 |
|---|---|---|

**Ingredients:**

- ¼ cup extra virgin olive oil
- Ten chopped garlic cloves
- Two chopped yellow onions
- Two chopped carrots
- One sliced sweet potato
- Two sliced potatoes
- Salt
- 1 tsp coriander
- 1 tbsp Harissa spice
- 1 tsp cinnamon
- 2 cups tomatoes
- ½ tsp turmeric
- ½ cup chopped dried apricot
- 2 cups cooked chickpeas
- Handful fresh parsley leaves
- ½ cup vegetable broth
- 1 tbsp lemon juice

**Directions:**

- ❖ Sauté onions in heated olive oil at high flame for five minutes in a Dutch oven.
- ❖ Stir in veggies, salt, garlic, and spices. Mix well and cook for eight minutes over medium flame with constant stirring.
- ❖ Mix in broth, apricot, and tomatoes and cook for the next ten minutes.
- ❖ Reduce the flame and let it simmer for 25 minutes.
- ❖ Add chickpeas and cook for five minutes.
- ❖ Sprinkle parsley and lemon juice and mix well.
- ❖ Serve and enjoy it.

**Nutrition:** Calories: 448 kcal Fat: 18.4 g Protein: 16.9 g Carbs: 60.7 g Fiber: 24 g

## 240) ITALIAN-STYLE GRILLED BALSAMIC CHICKEN WITH OLIVE TAPENADE

| Preparation Time: 10 minutes | Cooking Time: 30 minutes | Servings: 2 |
|---|---|---|

**Ingredients:**

- Two boneless chicken breasts
- 1/4 cup olive oil
- 1/4 cup balsamic vinegar
- 1/8 cup garlic mustard
- 1.5 tbsp balsamic vinegar
- Three minced garlic cloves
- 1 tbsp lemon juice
- 1 tbsp chopped herbs of choice
- 1 tsp kosher salt
- 1/2 tsp black pepper

**Directions:**

- ❖ Combine garlic, balsamic vinegar, lemon juice, pepper, olive oil, herbs, salt, and mustard in a bowl. Add chicken and toss well to coat chicken.
- ❖ Set aside for three hours.
- ❖ Brush oil over chicken pieces and grill gates.
- ❖ Cook chicken on grill gates for ten minutes from both sides.
- ❖ Occasionally brush the chicken with marinade while grilling it.
- ❖ When marks appear over the chicken, shift the chicken to the grill gate's cooler side and cook there for 12 minutes.
- ❖ Again, shift the chicken to the heated side of the grill gate and cook for ten more minutes.
- ❖ Place the grilled chicken on a plate and cover to keep it warm.
- ❖ Serve and enjoy it.

**Nutrition:** Calories: 352 kcal Fat: 21 g Protein: 35 mg Carbs: 5 g Fiber: 1 g

## 241) ITALIAN LINGUINE AND ZUCCHINI NOODLES WITH SHRIMP

| Preparation Time: 20 minutes | Cooking Time: 20 minutes | Servings: 6 |
|---|---|---|

**Ingredients:**

- ✓ 2/3 cup extra virgin olive oil
- ✓ 1 lb shrimp
- ✓ Four minced garlic cloves
- ✓ Black pepper to taste •
- ✓ 12 oz wheat linguine
- ✓ kosher salt to taste
- ✓ 3 tbsp butter
- ✓ Three zucchinis
- ✓ One lemon zested
- ✓ 1 tsp red chili flakes
- ✓ 3 tbsp lemon juice
- ✓ A handful of chopped parsley
- ✓ 1/2 cup shredded Parmesan cheese

**Directions:**

- ❖ Add salt, garlic, shrimps, pepper, and olive oil. Toss well to coat evenly. Keep it aside.
- ❖ Pour water into a pot and add salt to it. Let it boil and cook linguine in boiling water. Drain linguine and set aside.
- ❖ Heat olive oil in a skillet over medium heat and cook shrimps in it for three minutes from both sides. Shift the cooked shrimps into the plate.
- ❖ Melt butter in the same pan and sauté garlic, lemon juice, chili flakes, and lemon zest for one minute.
- ❖ Pour in pasta water in another pan and cook for three minutes. Add zucchini noodles and cook for two minutes with constant stirring.
- ❖ Transfer the noodles to the garlic mixture pan. Add linguine and cheese. Toss well.
- ❖ Pour in more of the pasta water to make a sauce of the desired level.
- ❖ Add shrimp, zucchini, salt, and pepper, and mix well.
- ❖ You can spread more cheese if you like.
- ❖ Garnish with parsley and serve.

**Nutrition:** Calories: 521 kcal Fat: 22 g Protein: 28 g Carbs: 52 g Fiber: 4 g

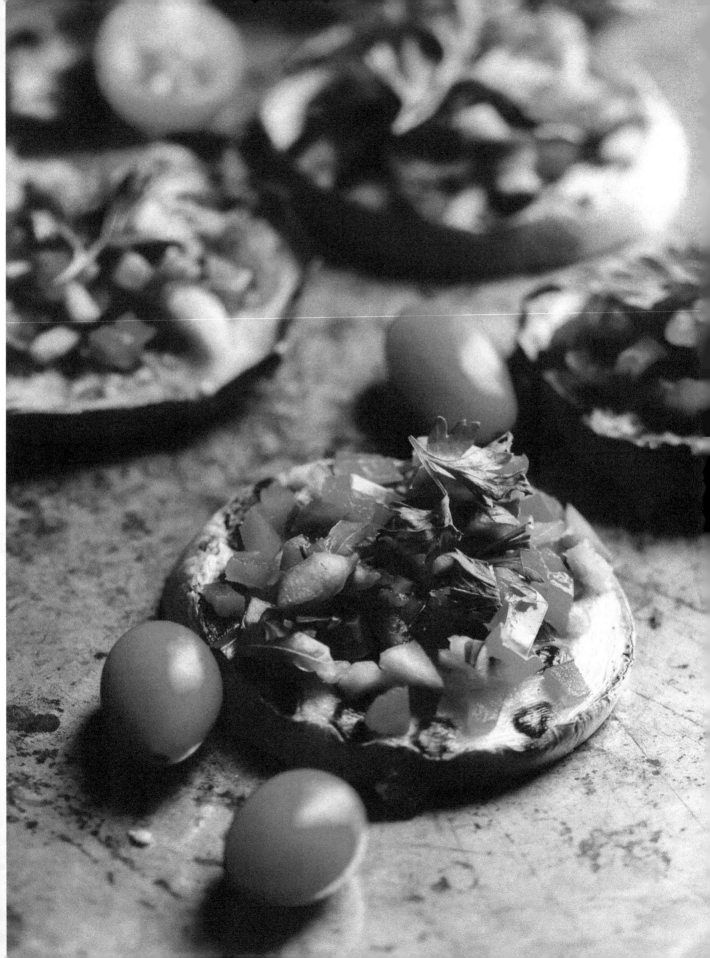

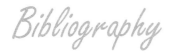
*Bibliography*

## FROM THE SAME AUTHOR

**ITALIAN COOKBOOK FOR ONE** - More than 120 Very Easy Recipes for Beginners! Delight yourself like in a restaurant with the best meals for weight loss and heart health!

**ITALIAN DIET FOR BEGINNERS** *Cookbook* - 120+ Super Easy Recipes to Start a Healthier Lifestyle! Discover the tastiest Diet overall to lose weight and stay Healthy!

**ITALIAN DIET FOR MEN** *Cookbook* - More than 120 seafood, vegetarian and meat recipes from the Best Mediterranean Cuisine! Stay FIT and HEALTHY with the perfect diet to lose weight before summer!

**ITALIAN DIET FOR WOMEN** *Cookbook* - The Best 120+ recipes for weight loss and stay HEALTHY! Maintain FIT your body and delight yourself with the best diet overall for heart health!

**ITALIAN DIET FOR KIDS** *Cookbook* - The Most Delicious 120 Recipes for Children, tested BY Kids FOR Kids! Stay FIT and HEALTHY with many seafood and vegetarian meals, HAVING FUN as in a restaurant!

**ITALIAN COOKBOOK FOR TWO** - The Best 220+ Seafood and Vegetarian Recipes For Mum and Kids! Stay HEALTHY and lose weight preparing these delicious meals with your family!

**ITALIAN COOKBOOK FOR COUPLE** - 220+ Delicious Recipes to make together! Eat with your Partner as in a Restaurant with the most complete guide about the Italian Cuisine for two!

**ITALIAN COOKBOOK FOR BEGINNER CHEF** - More than 220 Very Easy Recipes to Start your Italian Restaurant Cuisine! Delight yourself and your Friends with the Best Mediterranean Meals like a Chef!

**ITALIAN COOKBOOK FOR MEDITERRANEAN ATHLETES** - The Best 220+ Seafood and Vegetarian Recipes for Weight Loss and Heart Health! Stay FIT and LIGHT with The Most Delicious Diet Overall!

# Conclusion

Thanks for reading *"Italian Diet for Couple Cookbook"*!

I hope you liked this Cookbook and I wish you to achieve all your goals!

*Olivia Rossi*

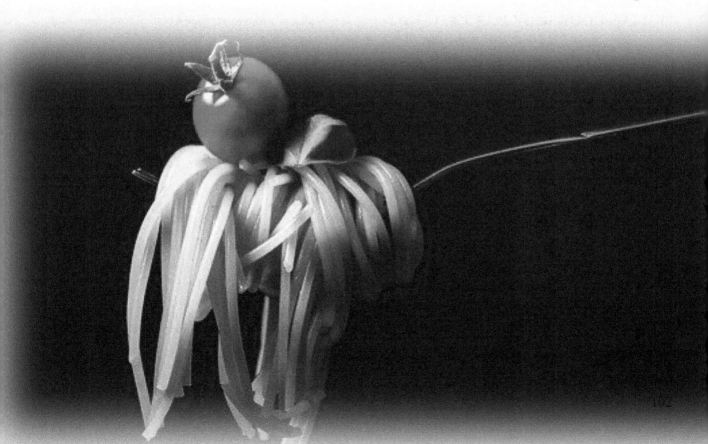

CPSIA information can be obtained
at www.ICGtesting.com
Printed in the USA
BVHW062126240521
607998BV00010B/1439